Are you overweight?

Do you feel unhealthy?

Do you feel tired?

Do you feel lethargic?

Do you feel depressed?

Are you overwhelmed, stressed
and lack the time to workout?

Frustrated with diets and the lack of results?

Have you lost and gained weight?

Confused about how to lose
the weight once and for all?

WE HAVE THE SOLUTION!

We will hand you the blueprint
to success. Walk through our doors
and we'll take care of the rest!

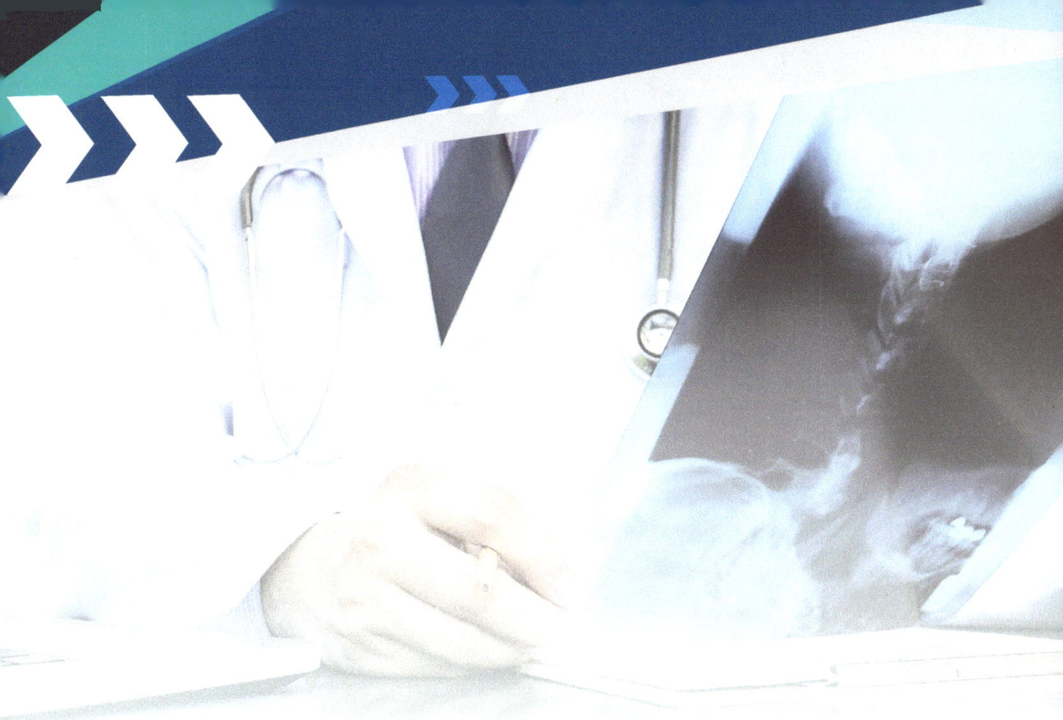

Why do we as Americans have THE HIGHEST RATES of degenerative disease than any industrialized country in the world?

If we have the best Health Care System in the world, then why are we so UN-healthy?

Let's look at some stats!

America is the richest nation in the world but embarrassingly enough we rank:

- **Infant Mortality: 33rd out of 36 industrialized nations**
- **Obesity- 36th out of 36 or DEAD LAST!**
- **Life Expectancy- 26th**

The total cost of Cardiovascular Disease in 2011 was 116.8 Billion dollars and this accounted for 36.5% of all total cardiovascular disease costs.

A whopping 62% of adults 65-74 have high blood pressure that puts them at risk for at least one form of cardiovascular disease.

These numbers equate to out of 85.6 million adults, 1 out of 3 people having one or more types of cardiovascular disease.

What about Cancer?
No better here.

In 2018 more then 1.7 million cases of cancer were diagnosed and as a result over 600,000 people died.

How about Diabetes?

Diabetes happens to be the 7th leading cause of death contributing to both Heart Disease and Stroke with an estimated cost of $327 billion dollars in 2017.

The saddest thing about our most common diseases is that they are totally preventable.

Could it be that "healthy eating" is making us sick? There are many reasons why we as Americans, the most industrialized nation in the world are so un-healthy, but the main reason could simply be that we are INDUSTRIALIZED.

This isn't necessarily a bad thing, right? I mean, I don't think you would enjoy performing hard labor everyday as people did in 18th and early 19th century. Americans have always taken the path of least resistance; by becoming more industrialized we have become more technological. By becoming more technological we have been able to get more work done in a shorter amount of time without expending too much energy. Try working for 8-12 hours a day standing up. It's not a coincidence that we are almost always sitting down to work.

So, technology in short has enabled us to invent, produce and sell "things" pretty much 24 hours a day.

That's quite a demand to keep up! This is part of my point. The "demand" to keep up with the economy and keeping your job forces people to work longer, sometimes to the affect of taking up a second job. This "demand" forces many parents to work outside

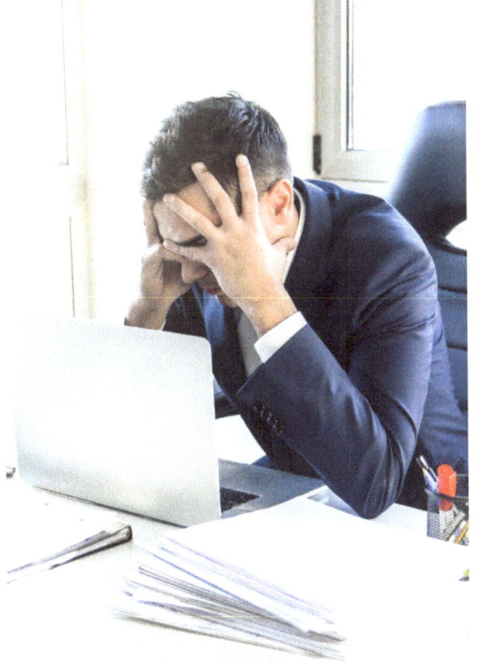

of the house, which leaves children, at home to feed and parent themselves.

With both parents working long hours and sometimes two and three jobs, what kind of time does that leave for cooking quality food for themselves and their kids? Parents arrive home exhausted from keeping up the high production and the "demand" from their employers to make more (services and money). This not only leaves a "demand" for the parents to find cheaper and faster ways to eat but also the children have to do the same thing.

So, in comes the processed food industry to save the day! TECHNOLOGY has allowed us to produce foods that have a long shelf-life (you don't have to cook them), these foods happen to be cheap, taste good and they can be eaten quickly.

The fact that these cheap/highly-processed foods are dead empty calories that have almost no nutritional quality is a major problem. These products are in "high demand" because we don't have time to cook. You must understand that if there is a "demand" for ANYTHING, someone is going to capitalize on it. We can argue that McDonald's and General Mills add things to their foods in order for you to get addicted (they do!) but neither of these company's forces anyone to eat it.

From a health stand point this is a vicious cycle that leads to:

1. Stress- As if you didn't have enough from the traffic on the way to work! This is a killer in of itself and I will delve into this subject thoroughly very soon.

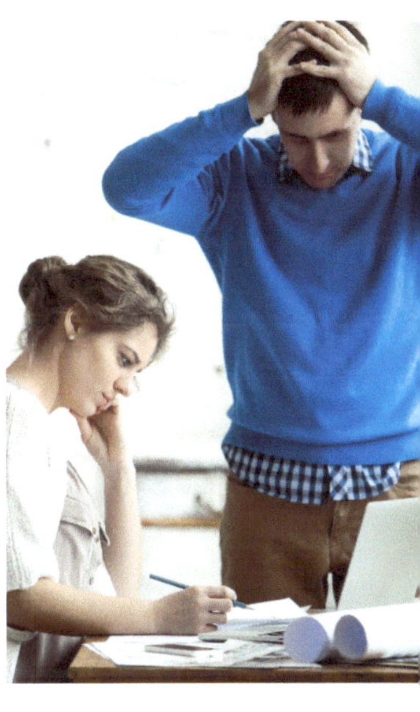

2. Lethargy- you're too tired to exercise and if you do have the energy you do something stupid like a spinning or aerobic class (more on that later).

3. Low Blood Sugar- Brain Fog and irritability occur and you make more poor food choices plus raise insulin levels and store body fat.

4. Symptoms- From headaches (migraines), stomach aches, rashes, colds/congestion, sleep disorders, sexual dysfunction, high blood pressure, blood sugar issues, abnormal cholesterol levels etc... I could go on for hours! But guess what? If you've got a symptom then "they've" got a remedy! Where there's a demand there's money and the Pharmaceutical companies are laughing all the way to the bank. Drugs are necessary no doubt but these drugs do more harm than good, trust me! The problem will still exist if not dealt with because what all drugs do is simply take care of the SYMPTOMS that your poor lifestyle is causing! They never address the underlying PROBLEM; they don't look for a cure, they just treat the SYMPTOM because there would be no more money if they found a cure.

I know it's hard to swallow... "What do you mean? Of course the medical industry is looking for a cure." It goes against human nature to believe that someone or an organization would care more about profits than your actual health and well-being. But we have to be honest with ourselves; the medical industry is a business. They have one obligation, just like any business and that is to make a profit! It is their legal obligation to their shareholders to increase SALES.

So, how much would the sales of a drug increase if a particular disease/symptom was eradicated or a cure was discovered? You got it! There isn't much of an incentive to cure anything. The ultimate goal of the Pharmaceutical Industry is to keep people alive but SICK! They don't want you dead, but then again they don't want you healthy either. Somewhere in between is perfect, that way you'll be a long-standing customer forever.

Disease- Breast Cancer, Heart Disease, Osteoporosis, Diabetes etc. Contrary to what your Health Care, I mean Sick Care provider told you these are all degenerative diseases caused by trashing your body with the foods that you demand.

I know, I know, it runs in the family... It's your genetics... Repeat after me, "Genetics loads the gun and LIFESTYLE pulls the trigger". Let's get into this further but first I need to let you know something very important.

Dear Busy Professional, It's not your fault...

The problem with fitness and nutrition advice these days is that one, there is an over-abundance of info, which often leads to confliction, frustration and eventual failure and two the majority of advice passed out is outdated, overly complicated and too difficult to sustain over the long-term.

Our goal with this book is to simplify your path to health by giving you simple tips and techniques that will lead to powerful yet sustainable results. We will then dispel some common myths that often prevent or hold people back from receiving their full potential.

By having the 5 my "5 Pillars" at your disposal you will finally have all the necessary tools needed to become the STRONGEST and healthiest version of yourself.

Let's start by getting our mind "right"!

We often see people setting themselves up for failure by simply possessing the wrong mindset.

Please know that without the right mindset you cannot effectively change your diet, show up at the gym or make any sort of positive changes to your long-term health.

Mindset matters most! Let's show you how your thoughts are actually the key to your success.

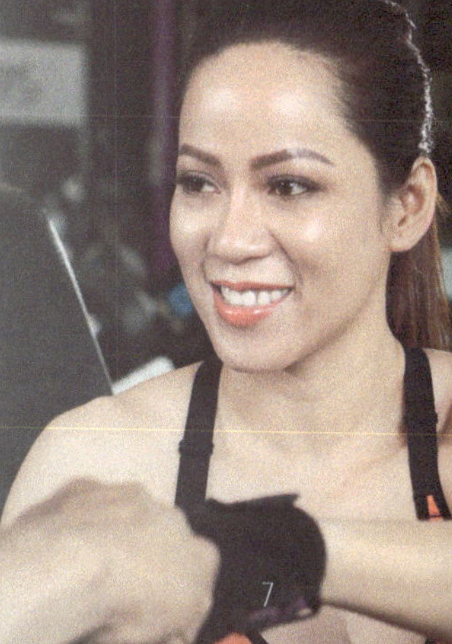

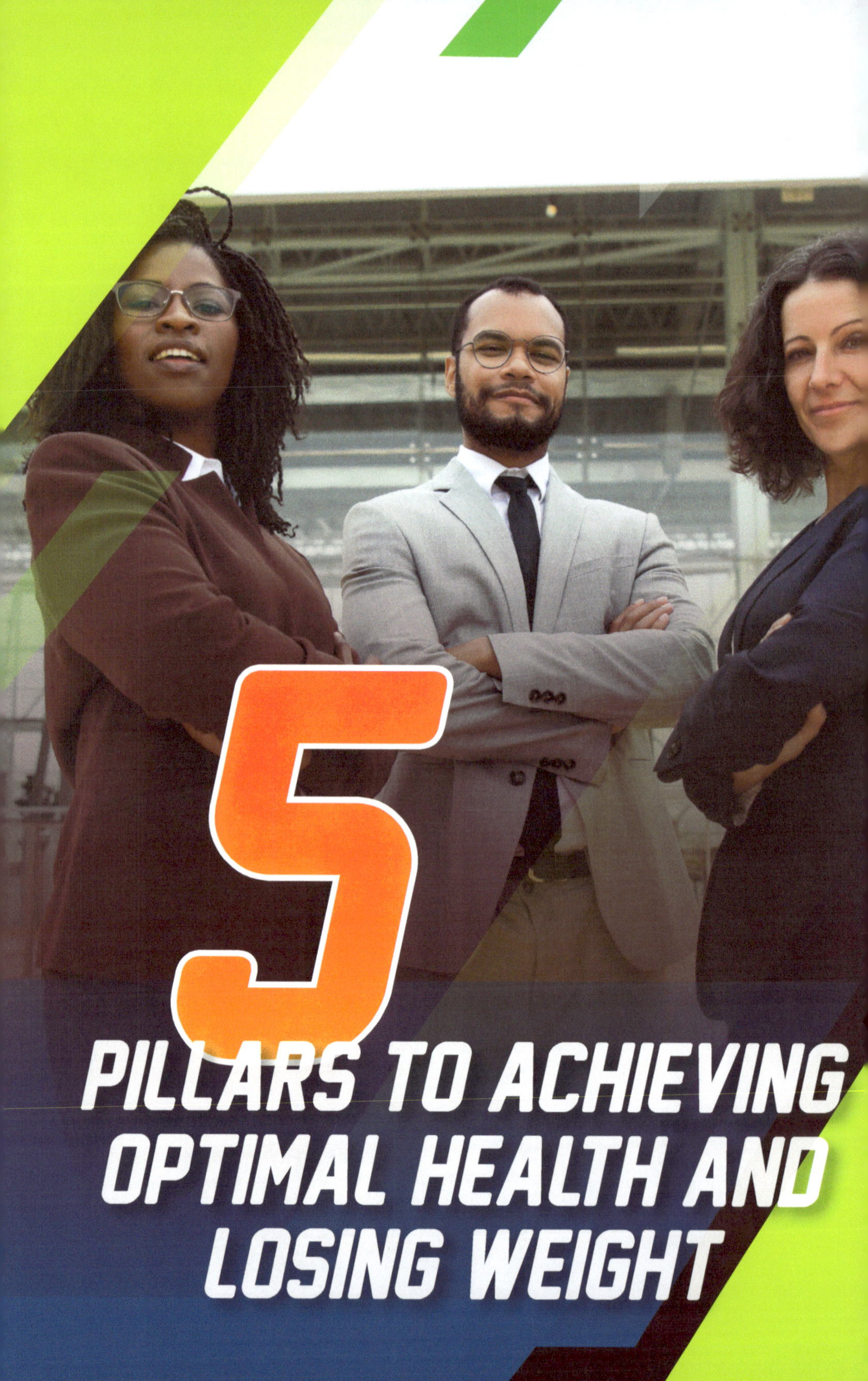

5
PILLARS TO ACHIEVING
OPTIMAL HEALTH AND
LOSING WEIGHT

MINDSET

Law of attraction- Energy Flows where energy goes

What are you thinking about? Where are your thoughts going? Are you focusing on what you don't want more of or focusing on what you do want more of? I think that's an important question to ask a lot of people. Because most people are saying, "Hey, I'm tired of being fat. I'm tired of being overweight. I'm tired of being broke. I'm tired of having bad relationships.. Why does this keep happening to me?"

These are negative thoughts that creep into the psyche unconsciously mostly at times. Your unconscious is a problem. So we need to start changing that mindset around what you want more of. When it comes to fat loss, forget thinking about fat. Going forward, let's focus on health and as a byproduct of you getting healthy you will in fact achieve what you really want which is fat loss or fitting in that size eight, or getting back in that dress, or fitting in those jeans that you always wanted to get back in, right? That's what you really want. Lets shift our energy and focus on what you want MORE of not the things that you'd like to do without.

S.M.A.R.T Goals

Before we jump in let's get some clarity on exactly what it is that you want to achieve. Setting goals is super important but first we have to make sure that they are
"S.M.A.R.T."

SMART is an acronym coined by Brian Tracy that stands for Specific Measureable Achievable Relevant and Timely.

S Specific- write out clear, concise goals

M Measurable- the ability to track your progress

A Achievable- set challenging yet achievable goals

R Relevant- set goals that are relevant to your overall life plan

T Timely- goal has a target finish time.

The "One Thing" is a fantastic book written by Gary Keller where he explains that it's not the actual goals that are most important. It's actually the ONE thing or "action" that needs to be taken to help you achieve the determined goals.

"What's the ONE thing I can do such that by doing it everything else will be easier or unnecessary."

In other words, what is the ONE thing that would have the biggest impact on you reaching your goal if NOTHING else changed?

So let's now go create your SMART goals and identify what the ONE thing would be to help you achieve your goals in a timely manner.

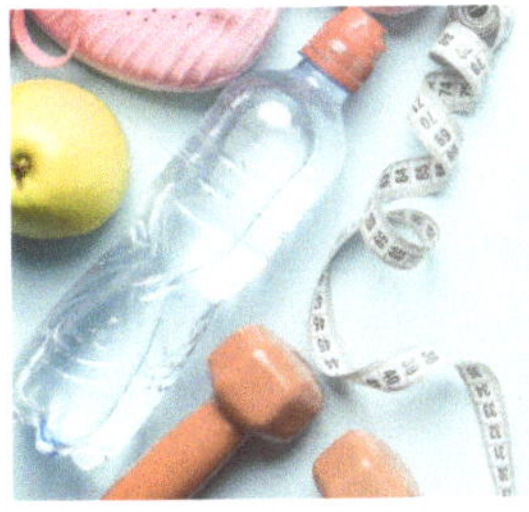

Now it's time to get your mind right and start putting your thoughts and energy into what you want more of.

You're going to create your new reality. I want you to visualize what you're asking for. See yourself leaner, healthier and stronger. How does it make you feel? It should feel FANTASTIC! Now ask yourself "why does it feel so good? From now on you stop saying, "I hope" and replace that with "I am".

You will start saying, "I am whatever I want or want to achieve."

> I'm so grateful that I'm healthy.
> I'm so grateful I'm strong.
> I'm so grateful I have so much energy.

You will start to live and act the person you want to be.

You will see, feel, hear, smell and touch everything that you desire as if you have already attained it.

Perception is reality and you will no longer accept your current state of reality, as you will create a new one. Having "laser focused mindset" such as this is KEY to attaining your SMART goals and focusing on your ONE Thing. I know this concept sounds weird or "Hokie Pokie" but how many times have you tried and failed in the past?

It's time for a paradigm shift!

We are taking you down a new road, one you probably have never traveled.

Why?

You've been down the other roads already and they all led you to a dead end.

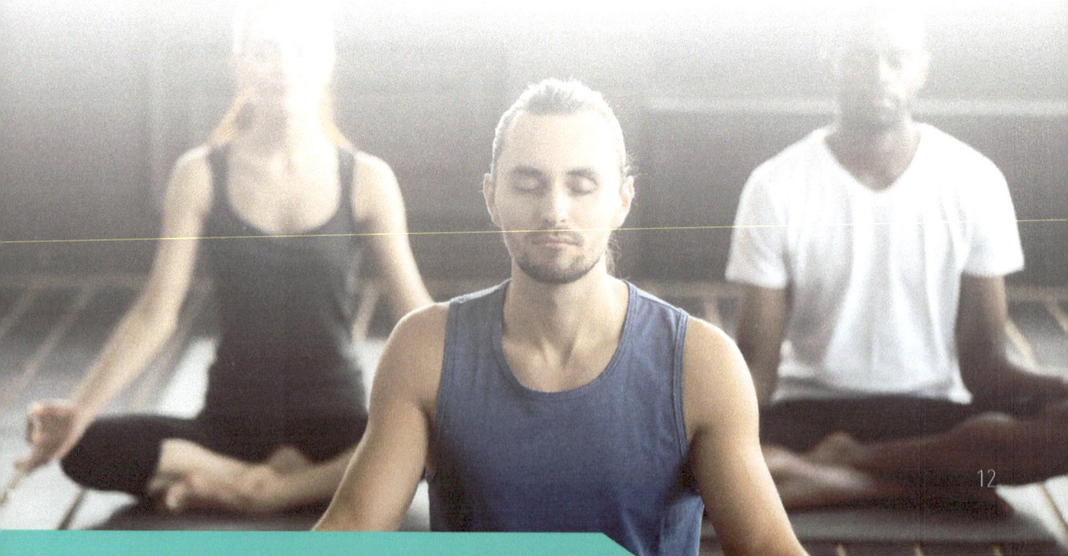

MOVEMENT

The Problem

Sitting—or just standing—kills and MOVEMENT heals.

We live in a society that makes it very easy to move less and burn less energy. It should be no wonder why the United States is the fattest and sickest country on the planet. We eat too much and the opportunities to sit on our butt are everywhere.

Katy Bowman, author of Move Your DNA states, "Although we're pretty proud of ourselves if we crank out 300 minutes of exercise per week, back in the day, our hunter-gatherer ancestors would move up to 8 hours a day or 3,000 minutes per week." So what types of movement are you engaging in when you're not exercising? Does your day look like this? You wake up early to bust out an awesome 60-minute workout then you:

- Sit in your car on the way to work
- Sit at your desk while at work
- Sit in your car coming home from work
- Sit at the dinner table to eat
- Sit on your couch and watch TV

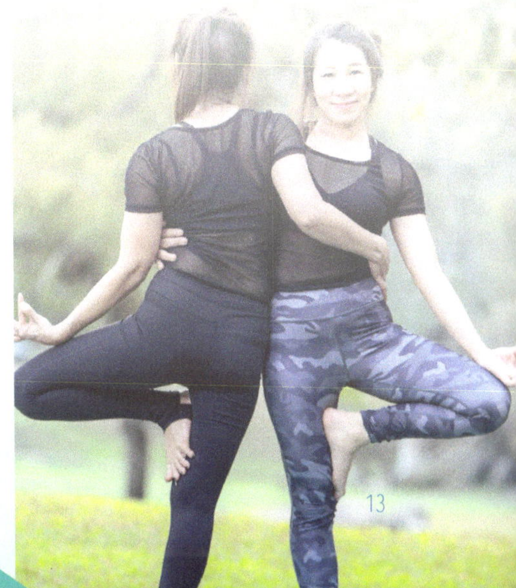

We shouldn't wonder why we have an obesity epidemic when we spend the majority of our time seated and sedentary. You are in fact seated the majority of your day and the majority of your life. So, put that in context, or perspective with how much you're actually working out percentage wise per week.

The bottom line is that people put way too much emphasis on exercising and working out. Working out alone just isn't as effective as most people think, and I'm going to prove it right now. Let's do some basic math shall we?

How many hours in a week? 168 correct?

Let's say you're working out five days a week for one hour. That's five hours of exercise per week. So what are you doing with the other 163 hours of the week? More than likely you are sitting at your desk or in your car.

There is no amount of working out that can compete with the amount of time we are not moving. We just can't compete with the inactivity.

We have to be honest and admit that working out is just the "icing on the cake", and the actual "cake" is movement and nutrition the two most important factors to long-term health and the actual solution to the obesity problem we are currently dealing with.

"Exercise is to movement
what a multivitamin is to food."

Don't make the common mistake of substituting moving for working out. Exercise should complement daily movement like a multivitamin should complement a quality diet.

Let's get our "NEAT" on!

N-E-A-T. or Non Exercise Activity Thermogenesis. NEAT is the amount of movement that you're getting in throughout your day while NOT exercising. Getting your NEAT on options could be:

- Walking around the office
- Walking your dog
- Just being "fidgety"
- Stretching/mobility

A great way to track NEAT would be to purchase and wear a pedometer and work toward getting in 10,000 steps per day. Add the 10,000 steps in per day along with exercising two or three days a week and were "moving" in the right direction.

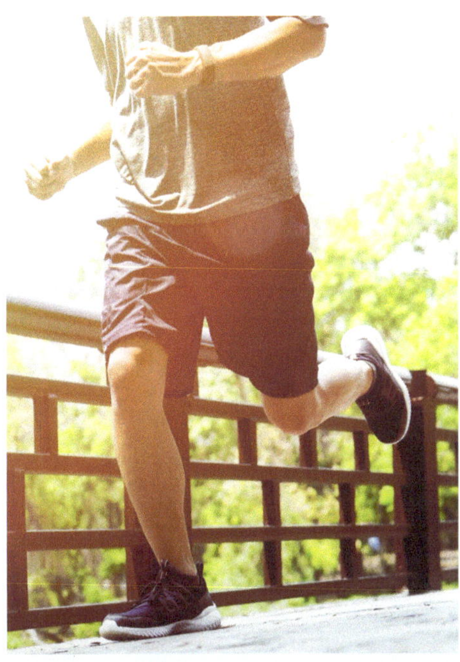

NUTRITION

There are many problems with mainstream diets and weight loss programs, but they all have one thing in common.

They are usually temporary and set the user up for eventual failure and weight gain.

Will such diets work?

Absolutely they'll work if you're able to stay with them long enough to see the results.

Here in lies the problem. Diets that require long-term restriction are simply not sustainable over the long term.

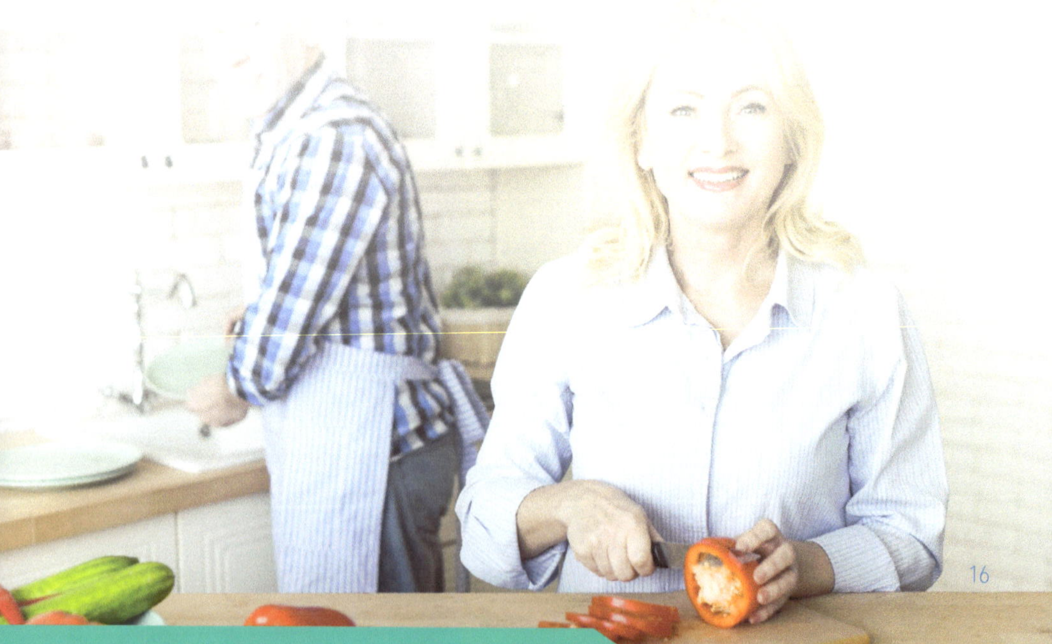

In my experience, most people fail to achieve long-term health and weight loss for one of the three reasons below:

- ▸ You either lose the weight crazy fast using pills, shakes, detoxes and prepackaged meals to find out it's not realistic to maintain and it's simply not sustainable so you quit and gain the weight back.

- ▸ You lose the weight so slow by restricting entire food groups or foods that you love. By the time you get to your goal, you realize you can't maintain the restriction and you finally realize that the lifestyle isn't sustainable, so you quit and gain the weight back.

- ▸ You get the meal plan from the nutritionist or dietician that requires you count calories, measure and weigh your foods and cook in bulk. You soon realize the amount of money you're spending on food, the time away from your family and friends due to cooking, the lack of production at work because you're eating all the time only to realize, you guessed it...

You can't maintain the restriction, the time, the money and realize that it's not sustainable so you quit and gain the weight back.

Does this sound familiar?

Tried some of these approaches before?

Which one of these categories are you in?

The bottom line is that all diets and approaches work as long as you're in a caloric deficit.

Calories are KING and there is no way around that.

Calories are KING!

No matter what diet you're on, whether it's ketogenic or whether it is vegan, you have to be in a caloric deficit to lose weight but let's make this even simpler…

Now, when it comes to meals, typical advice given, the common advice given to most Boomers and busy professionals is that you must eat a certain amount of calories per day by eating small meals every two to three hours. You're more than likely also told that you must cook in bulk and have your food prepared for the week and don't forget you must weight and measure each meal before being eaten too…

This is standard advice given by nutritionists, body builders and trainers but I have one question to ask you.

How's that working for you out there?

The Current Recommended Model Is Broken is:

- Too Complicated
- Too Confusing
- Too Time Consuming
- Too Costly
- Unrealistic
- Unsustainable

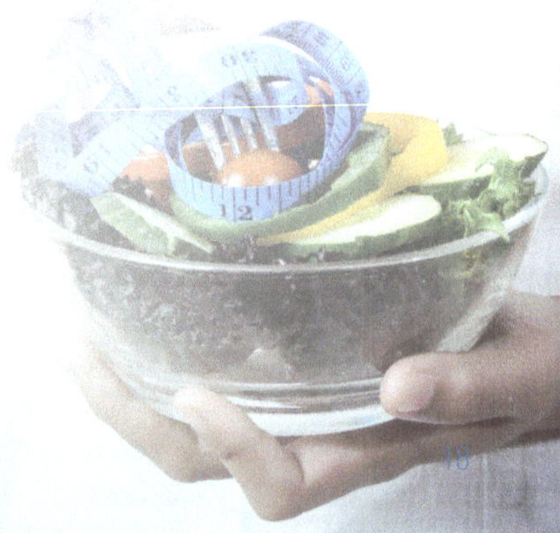

Now if this model is currently working for you then I think you should keep doing it. But if it's not sustainable and it's not working for you then it's time for something different.

I've found over the last 20 years and working with 1000's of client's that the easiest and most bang for your buck change that can be made is to "JERF" or just eat real food.

Are there other things that we can implement? Of course but this is the ONE thing that can have the biggest impact on your health without anything else changing. Heard that phrase before?

"Just eating real food" or "JERF" simply means eating foods closest to their natural state. These are foods that have no more than one ingredient and can usually be found on the perimeter of the grocery store or market. If the food you'd like to consume comes in a box, were going to limit that consumption. If that food has a shelf life, meaning it will NOT go bad or spoil were going to limit that consumption.

In other words, were going to choose to consume REAL food.

Just eating REAL food alone will accomplish many things:

- You'll consume less calorie's
- You'll consume higher quality food's
- You'll have less sweet cravings
- You'll be more satiated
- Your health will improve
- You'll have Increased energy levels
- You'll lose weight
- You'll have better quality skin
- You'll have improved quality of sleep
- You'll have improved mental clarity
- You'll have less inflammation

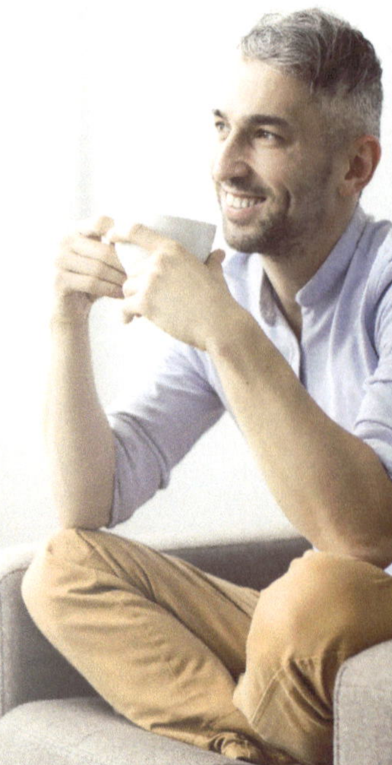

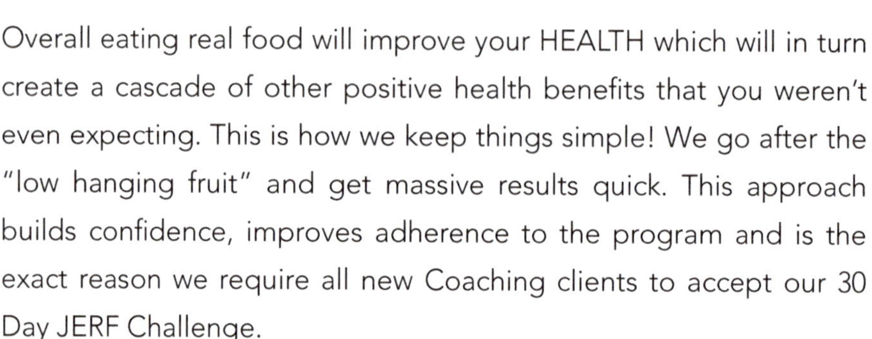

Overall eating real food will improve your HEALTH which will in turn create a cascade of other positive health benefits that you weren't even expecting. This is how we keep things simple! We go after the "low hanging fruit" and get massive results quick. This approach builds confidence, improves adherence to the program and is the exact reason we require all new Coaching clients to accept our 30 Day JERF Challenge.

The results that we routinely see from changing food quality alone are life-changing. See our testimonial section for others we've worked with.

Eliminating Meals vs Decreasing Calories or JERF on Steroids

The next most important thing in our quest for optimal health and losing body fat will be to implement yet another simple yet POWERFUL technique that gets you to eat less calories without actually counting calories or measuring the amount of food you take in each meal.

Instead of calorie restriction we will use MEAL restriction or something that I call Time Restricted Eating. It's just semantics right?

I mean, it's all the same thing in the long run. We know that calories are KING and that in order for you to lose weight there must be a caloric deficit but why must the deficit come from counting calories and measuring food portions? How about we accomplish the needed calorie deficit from reducing meals instead?

By reducing meals we reduce calories but without the tedious counting of calories. Going forward you will eat 2-3 meals per day, sometimes less but no more then 3. By eliminating snacking and decreasing meal frequency we will effectively do the following:

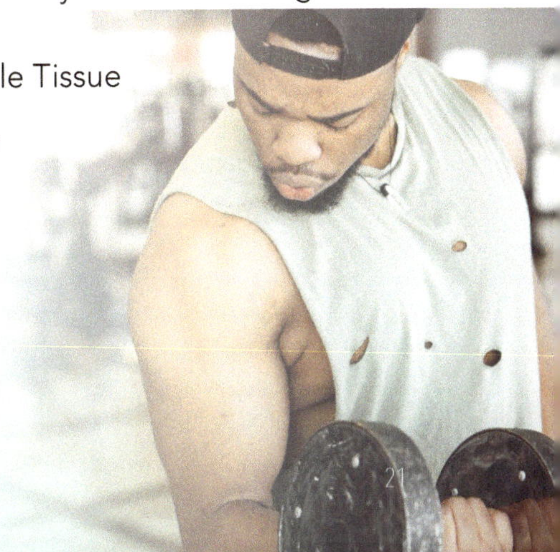

- Helps Body Maintain Lean Muscle Tissue
- Help Eliminate Food Addictions
- Improve Gut Health
- Improve Lipid Panel
- Improved Sleep
- Reduce Alzheimer's risk

It's a very simple tactic but right now most people have been brainwashed into thinking they need to eat multiple meals per day and snack in between. Some people are even told that the reason that they're over-weight is because they aren't eating enough?? Crazy right?

The bottom line is that losing weight is simple. It's not always easy but in my 20yr experience there's isn't anything easier or more sustainable then eating real food and decreasing meal frequency aka. Time Restricted Eating or Increasing the amount of time in between meals.

The Powerful Benefits of Time-Restricted Eating

- Increases Lifespan- Great effect on autophagy (process by which a cell recycles itself to make sure that it can function the best it can by getting rid of anything that isn't working properly
- Increases Body's Resistance to Stress
- Improves Brain Function
- May aid in preventing Cancer
- Improves Immune System
- Improves Insulin Sensitivity
- Better Heart Health
- Lower Inflammation
- Raises Growth Hormone Levels
- Helps in Weight Loss
- Helps Clear Skin & Prevent Acne
- Lowers Risk of Deadly Diseases

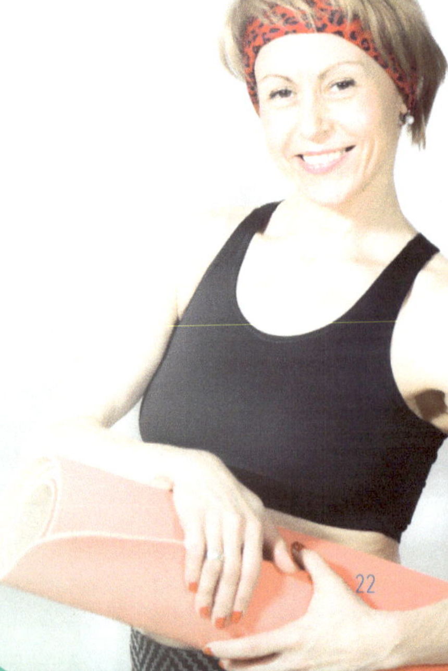

Let's do some more math…

We already have determined that calories are KING and in order for us to lose weight we must be in a caloric deficit. Let's assume that you are over-weight with a a goal of losing and you communicate to me that you are eating 3 main meals (breakfast, lunch and dinner) with two snacks (mid-morning and mid-afternoon). The total amount of meals per week would be 35 correct?

My advice right off the bat would be to eliminate the mid-morning and mid-afternoon snacks. This is a simple change and will lower are meal frequency from 35 meals per week to 21 meals per week. Baring that this person isn't eating and drinking everything but the kitchen sink over the weekend, shouldn't this person lose weight with a meal reduction of 14 meals?

Let's go even further. This person has lost 10 pounds just by eliminating snacks and decreasing his/her meals by 14. I think you can see where I'm going with this but now imagine that this person was JERF?

Are you going to lose weight? Yep, unless you mess it up on the weekend or make up for it somewhere else. But that's a huge caloric deficit right there. Are you going to die? No. Are you in danger? No. There's nothing wrong with skipping meals. There's no science that says you have to eat breakfast, eat every 2-3 hours or three square meals a day for that matter. If you're eating all the time, you're simply impairing your ability to get healthy and lose weight.

Cut the meals and you end up cutting the calories.

More Advantages to Eating Fewer Meals

- It's simple

- It's FREE

- It's convenient

- Enjoy life's little pleasures

- It's POWERFUL

- It's flexible

- It works with ANY diet

- It's HEALTHY

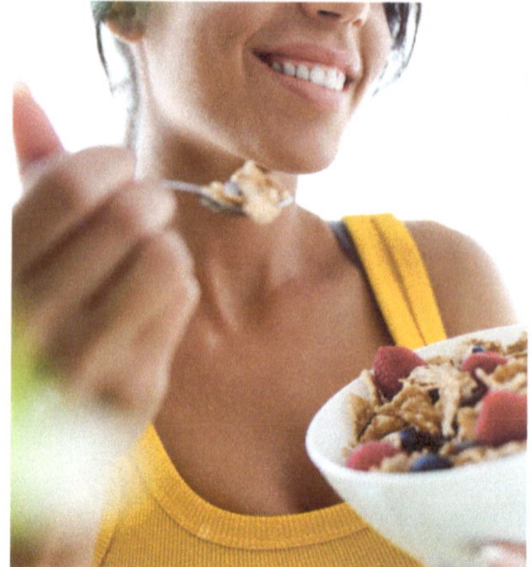

Why is it that I'm constantly seeing overweight people in the gym that workout seven days a week?

I see overweight people that finish marathons.
I see over-weight spinning and aerobic instructors.
I see overweight people on Vegan Diets and see over-weight people on the Keto Diet and Paleo Diets.

All these people have ONE thing in common.

They are eating too many calories.

The marathon runner can't out run a caloric surplus. The spinning and aerobic instructor can't out exercise a caloric surplus and the person on the Vegan diet is consuming too many calories coming from Vegetables, Fruits and Grains while the people on the Keto and Paleo diet are consuming too many calories from Protein and Fat.

There is no magic diet or no amount of exercise that can un-do this and you can't workout longer or more often.

The only logical thing to do is to take in less calories and the easiest way to take in less calories is by consuming less MEALS.

So I challenge you to stop counting calories, JERF and start eliminating meals.

You will not only lose weight from using this tool but more importantly you will be healthier which is the most important anyways.

Living this type of lifestyle you will actually save money, have more time, get healthier, lose fat, and most importantly you will have the motivation to keep the weight you lost off FOREVER!

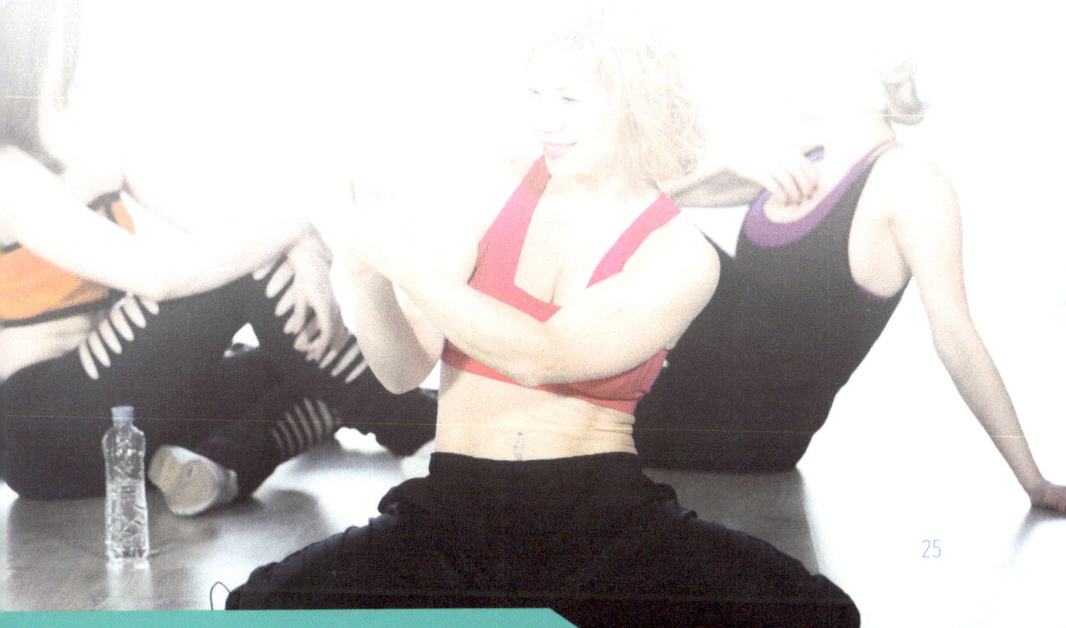

MATT'S 10 RULES OF NUTRITIONAL SUCCESS

RULE 1: Eat no more than three meals per day (STOP SNACKING!)

At each of those meals make sure you eat a protein and plenty of vegetables. Save carbs for days that you exercise and earn those carbs.

RULE 2: Boxed food in moderation.

If the food product is found in a box or has an expiration date, then it should be eaten in moderation.

RULE 3: What not to buy.

If the food product contains high fructose corn syrup, MSG, partially hydrogenated anything, food colorings, or a substance that you can't pronounce, do not purchase or eat that product! Also stay away from any product that says low-fat or that makes other health claims. Low-fat means high sugar. If it's too good to be true, it probably is.

RULE 4: Shop the perimeters.

The bulk of the food items in your grocery cart should be coming from the perimeter of the grocery store. This means meats, vegetables, fruits, seeds (sunflower, pumpkin, etc.), raw nuts (cashews, pecans, walnuts, almonds, Brazil nuts), real eggs, butter, and full-fat dairy products.

RULE 5:   Don't drink your calories.

The majority of your beverage consumption should be coming from non-caloric drinks such as water. Try to only purchase water out of a glass. Water found in plastic bottles/containers has been exposed to high heat either through transportation or different forms of storage. This high heat causes plastic to leak phytoestrogens into the water. When consumed, these estrogens cause hormonal imbalances and many other health related problems.

RULE 6:   Strive to only purchase organic, hormone-free, antibiotic-free meat products.

Better yet, support your local farmers market and buy grass-fed animal products. Grass is a natural diet for animals. Grass-fed animals have a much higher ratio of Omega 3:6 fatty acids versus corn-fed animals. Animal products sold in your local grocery store are fed corn and other grains—an unnatural diet that makes animals sick. This is why they are pumped full of antibiotics that are ultimately being eaten by you, the consumer. Besides being pumped full of antibiotics, these animals are also given hormones to make them grow faster and weigh more. Again, as a consumer of these animal products, you are eating what the animal ate.

Lastly, local groceries are selling cruelly treated animals that never see the light of day. You can bypass this problem and help support the fair treatment of animals by refusing to purchase animal products from traditional grocery stores. Stick to places that offer organic, humanly-treated, antibiotic-free, hormone-free, grass-fed animal products. Even better, seek out a local farmer's market or farm to support their hard work and dedication.

RULE 7:   **Find affordable ways to eat healthy.**

I realize that choosing higher quality food is more expensive. If you can't afford to buy all organic or from a farmer's market, I highly suggest that you buy vegetables and fruits from your local grocery store to save some money. Why only buy meat from the farmer's market? There are methods of washing pesticides and herbicides off your fruits and veggies, but it is impossible to eliminate the toxins found in meat products.

Therefore, if you are on a budget while trying to eat better quality foods, it's a better idea to split trips. It's a minor hassle but I highly recommend making one trip to local grocery for veggies and fruits followed by one trip to an organic market or farmer's market to purchase meats. Not only does this cut down on your food bill, but it also allows you to provide the healthiest food items to yourself and your family.

RULE 8:   **Spread the word.**

The more people we get the word out to about the benefits of purchasing organic, grass-fed animal products and pesticide-free vegetables, the more affordable they will become. Essentially, you're voting for the foods grocery stores make available and the pricing of those foods by shopping behavior. If your cart is filled with packaged, barcoded products with expiration dates, then you're asking for more of the same. Change your shopping tactics by making better, informed, healthy choices. This will lead to healthy goods being more affordable for everyone.

RULE 9: Plan ahead.

Prepare meals in advance to make sure you just aren't grabbing whatever is available. Make your healthy food what's easiest and available.

RULE 10: Plan to break the rules 10% of the time.

We like to advocate for the 90/10 rule. This means you should practice the first nine habits 90% of the time while allowing yourself to "break your diet" 10% of the time. Let's do some math. Let's say that you eat 3 times a day for a weekly total of 21 meals. According to our 90/10 rule, this allows you to partake in 2.1 "breaks" per week (or two cheat meals). For those two meals, eat whatever you desire. The important part is to remember, it's just two meals, not two days.

Remember, it's about health first. The healthier you are, the less body fat you will carry.

THE JERF30 FOOD LIST

		DO IT!	PASS IT UP!
Proteins and Fats	**PRIMARY PROTEINS/ FATS**	Bass, beef, bison, buffalo, chicken, clams, crayfish, duck, eggs with yolks, elk, emu, game hens, goose, grouse, halibut, lamb, lobster, mackerel, mahi mahi, mussels, mutton, organ meats, oysters, pork, rabbit, red snapper, salmon, sardines, scallop, tuna, trout, turkey, veal, venison, wild game	Lunch meats, hot dogs, any other processed meat, shark, swordfish, orange roughy (these fish are high in mercury), most protein powders (see page 81)
	FATS & OILS	Avocado, avocado oil (cold pressed), bacon fat, chicken fat, coconut butter, coconut milk, coconut oil, duck fat, flax oil (cold pressed), ghee, lard, olives, olive oil (cold pressed), tallow, sesame oil (cold pressed)	Canola oil, cottonseed oil, Crisco, hydrogenated oils, imitation butters (if it's not butter, then what the heck is it?), shortening, soybean oil, vegetable oil
	NUTS & SEEDS	Almonds, almond butter, brazil nuts, cashews, cashew butter, chestnuts, flax seeds, hazelnuts, macadamia nuts, peanuts, pecans, pine nuts, pistachios, pumpkin seeds, sesame seeds, sunflower seeds, walnuts Note: nuts should be preferably raw.	Roasted, salted, or sugar-coated nuts and seeds Note: If you have allergic reactions to nuts, please continue to avoid them.
	DAIRY	**(Avoid until after the 8th day)** raw butter, raw cheeses, raw cultured dairy products (kefir, yogurt), raw milk	All other organic or commercial dairy products, including butter
Carbohydrates	**VEGGIES**	**Low/Medium-Starchy Vegetables** (including but not limited to): Artichoke, asparagus, beet greens, broccoli, brussels sprouts, cabbage, carrots, cauliflower, cilantro, collards, cucumber, dandelion, eggplant, endive, green onions, kale, kohlrabi, lettuce, mushrooms, mustard greens, onions, parsley, peppers, radish, rutabaga, sea vegetables, spinach, swish chard, tomatillos, tomato, turnip greens, turnips, yellow squash, watercress, zucchini **Starchy Vegetables*** (including but not limited to): Beet, parsnip, pumpkin, sweet potatoes, winter squash, yams * Consume starchy vegetables in small amounts. They are best eaten directly after exercise.	
	FRUITS Limit fruit to 2-3 servings per day	(Including but not limited to): Apricot, berries of all types*, cantaloupe, casaba melon, cherries, coconut*, figs, grapefruit, grapes, guava, green apples*, honeydew melon, kiwi, kumquat, lemon, lime, mango, melon, nectarine, orange, papaya, passion fruit, peaches, pears*, persimmon, pineapple, plums, pomegranate, raisin, red apples * Indicates fruits that are lower in sugar and preferable for those seeking fat loss	Canned fruits
	SUGARS, FLOUR PRODUCTS, GRAINS, & BEANS	**Avoid them all as best as possible.** If you are having a tough time adjusting to this, small amounts of beans, rice, buckwheat, quinoa, millet, corn, and gluten-free oats are acceptable. Note: Stevia, xylitol, and unheated, unfiltered honey are acceptable in moderation.	
	BEVERAGES	Consume about half your body weight in ounces of filtered water daily, preferably between meals. For variety, have coconut water, herbal tea, and/or fresh vegetable or fruit juice.	

STRENGTH

Strength training is king if the goal is changing body composition, or aesthetics. It is king. It may not be glamorous; it may not be the go-to, the most popular trending thing. As a matter of fact, I think strength training is probably the ugly stepchild of the fitness industry at this current time.

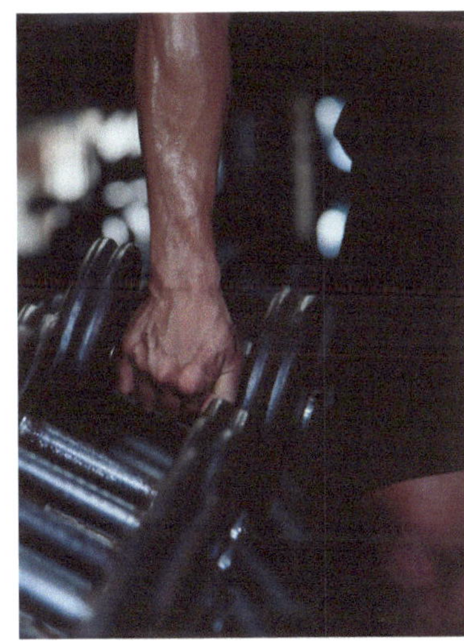

Cardio is just what's in, it's the most popular form of exercise and no one can deny that. Running long distance would have to take the cake for the most popular form of aerobics but we can't forget other hugely popular brands like Cross Fit, Orange Theory and Barry's Bootcamp, or Infomercials like P90X which seems to be found in every TV wall unit or side table collecting dust. Businesses and brands like these promote sweat, soreness and being tired to get results. I'm not at all saying that cardio isn't important, or it can't be part of your weekly routine. I'm saying it should complement a structured, progressive strength and conditioning workout and not be the all be all or sole modality that takes up your time.

I'm a big believer that strength training should be in your life at least twice a week, eight times a month. My friend Ben Bruno once stated that Strength Training should be your "main plate" while everything else like your aerobics classes, spinning, yoga, Pilates, Barre Class, boxing etc. should be considered "side dishes". I love this analogy and totally agree!

If the goal is changing your body composition, "toning up", getting "ripped or losing body fat then Strength Training should be a part of the weekly program but why?

Well, strength training or load bearing exercise builds muscle. You see, muscle tissue is considered "metabolically active tissue" meaning that the more muscle you have on your body, the more calories your body will expend at rest. So, while you're sitting in traffic, doing work at your desk or watching TV with your family that lean muscle that you earned through Strength Training 2-3X per week is burning calories while doing NOTHING. More importantly, load bearing exercise or Strength Training will help you get STRONGER which will allow you Boomers to play with your Grandchildren, carry groceries, walk up stairs and do all the things you'd like to do with less worry of injury.

Need more reason to Strength Train?

- Less risk of injury
- Improved bone density
- Improved lipid panel
- Improved hormonal panel
- Improved body composition

- Improved posture
- Increase muscle tone
- Increase confidence
- Decrease body fat
- Improve insulin sensitivity

And if the goal is aesthetics or you want to look better in your clothing, on the beach or with your partner of significant other then Strength Training beats cardio and the other "side dishes" here too.

Getting Stronger will also produce some other cool side effects like:

- Improved libido
- Running or jogging faster
- Stronger/stable Yoga poses
- Higher RPMs on that bike ride
- Longer runs with less risk of injury
- Clothes fitting better
- Improved endurance/lung capacity
- Increase in metabolic rate
- More reps with a heavier load
- Improved self-image

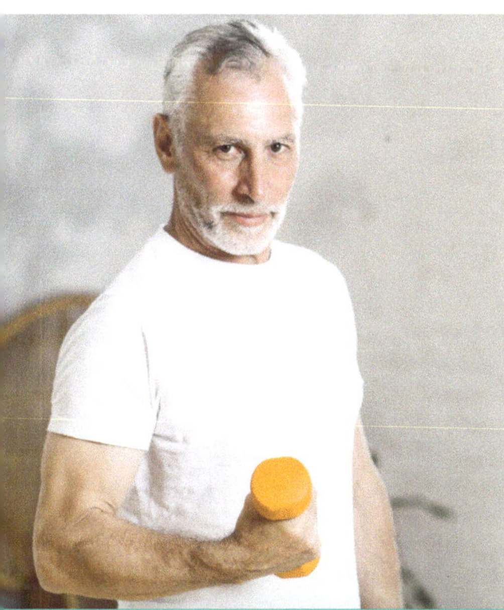

The bottom line is that if you have time for only one activity, choose Strength Training. It simply has more "bang for the buck" and when added to quality nutrition, less meals, adequate cardio program, quality sleep and stress management you are on your way to a long and prosperous life.

RECOVERY AKA. "WORKING IN"

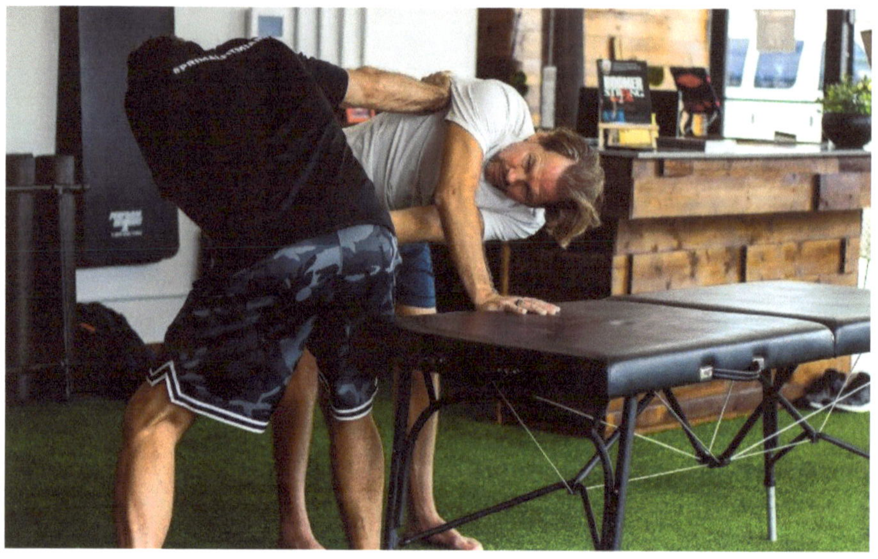

So, now that Dad and I have convinced you to MOVE throughout your day and were so happy that you're now working "OUT" getting at least two Strength Training sessions in per week but how are you working "IN"?

Going forward we want you to think of your body, that incredible vessel that you walk around in everyday as a "bank account". When you're moving or working out you are essentially spending "money"/ withdrawing funds or expending energy out of your bank account. Let's imagine that you're working out too much and you're limited on the amount of "funds" in your account/body. You know this term or scenario to be going into over-draft or bouncing a check but in my world we attribute your "lack of funds" to some sort of pain, or over-use injury.

Now we all know that the best way to prevent your bank account from going into over draft or bouncing a check would be to make a deposit right?

But what about your body?

How do we make a deposit or work "in" in order to prevent pain or worse a serious injury from taking place?

Here is a list of my 10 favorite ways to make a
Deposit into your "bank" aka. Your body:

1. Sleep
2. Meditation
3. Belly Breathing
4. Daily mobility- See morning ritual
5. JERF
6. Water intake (1/2 your bodyweight in ounces)
7. Stretching/massage
8. Yoga
9. Tai-chi
10. Cryotherapy

Let me stress that this list will serve you best if you make it a part of your week. You must be PRO-active vs being RE-active. Just as Dad and I stress the importance of preventing illness from occurring by using the 4 Pillars above our 5th Pillar Recovery works best when done on a DAILY basis to PREVENT an injury from occurring.

Don't make the mistake of doing what so many do and start using these techniques and modalities once you're already in pain. We highly suggest that you make daily deposits into your "bank account" so that you never have to worry about going into over-draft. Remember that in this case your over-draft fee won't be to your actual bank unfortunately the payment you'll be making will be to your orthopedic surgeon.

Now that we know the 5 Pillars to Boomer success let's go over your Blueprint to finding optimal health, moving better, feeling better and looking better.

The Busy Professional Blueprint to Success

1. Create your S.M.A.R.T Goals and determine your ONE Thing
2. Eat real food 90% of the time
3. Stop snacking and decrease meal frequency
4. MOVE at least 10,000 steps EVERYDAY
5. Workout ie. Strength Train at least 2X per week FOREVER.
6. Work "IN" DAILY to prevent pain and injury
7. Smile, hug, high five and give more then you receive

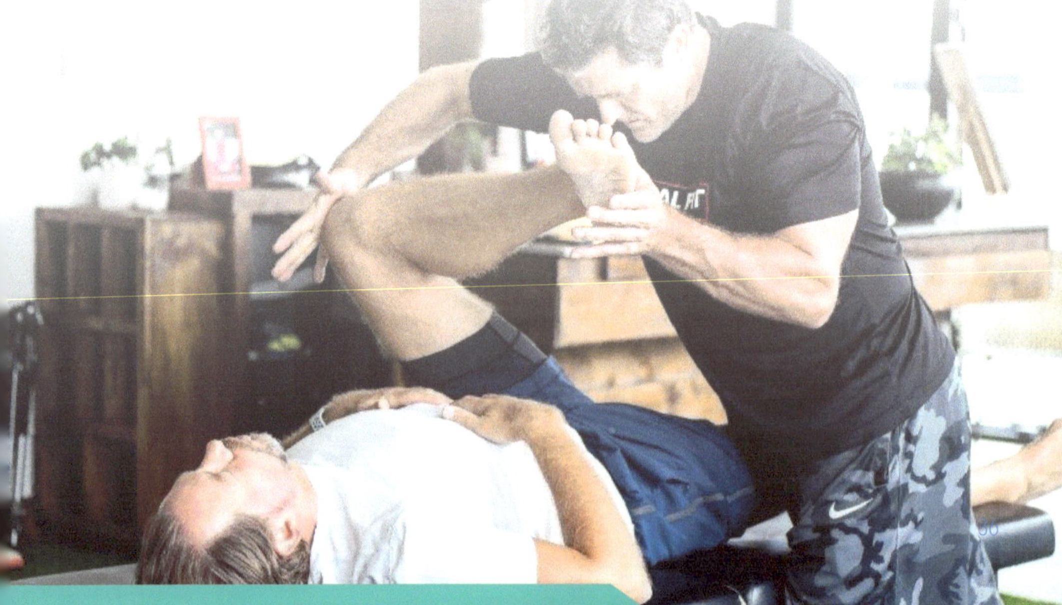

YOUR 30 DAY CHALLENGE

Are you ready to walk on the beach this summer confident and proud?

Ready to finally take control of your weight once and for all?

I invite you to go over to www.primalfit360miami.com/30/ and watch my Nutrition presentation.

During this 1hr Presentation you will learn exactly what I did to help a group of PF members lose over 100 pounds in 30 days!

In fact they each lost between 12-22 pounds each and we had 3 of them lose over 20 inches total in that 30 day span.

This info is so powerful yet so simple and I can't wait
to show you how to incorporate this tool into your life.

Some may be saying, "20 pounds in 30 days,
that's not realistic nor is it sustainable."

I beg to differ...

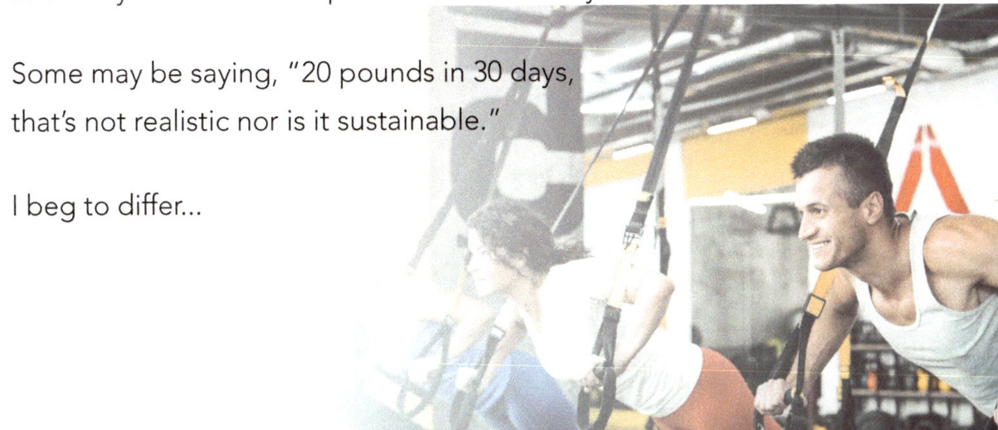

Let me explain.

The people I'm helping currently have battled weight most of there lives and have lost and gained weight more than they can remember.

In my experience most people have a negative relationship with food and some are more than likely dealing with food addictions.

Our program deals with these food relationships and empowers them to finally take control of eating once and for all.

Traditional diet programs can only promise on average 1-2 pounds per WEEK and SLOW weight loss like this though it's considered to be "normal" couldn't be more de-motivating especially when their is a significant amount of weight to lose.

I use to believe and "sell" this "slow and steady" way of weight loss but I'm now changing my mindset.

Nothing could be more frustrating then to workout so hard and invest so much so often to see lack luster results.

Enough Is enough!

The goal now is to take the weight off as quickly as possible and empower each of you to take massive action towards a healthier you.

Allow me to introduce you to a simple, effective and SUSTAINABLE tool that will officially end your weight loss challenges forever.

This program features a customized nutrition program and a private Facebook support group where you will be receiving coaching, accountability, and a blueprint to achieve optimal health and finally lose the weight as fast as possible.

This is NOT another diet!

This is a tool, but most importantly a sustainable way of life that works in conjunction with any diet or regimen you adhere to.

Will you join me on this 30-Day quest to discover the best version of yourself?

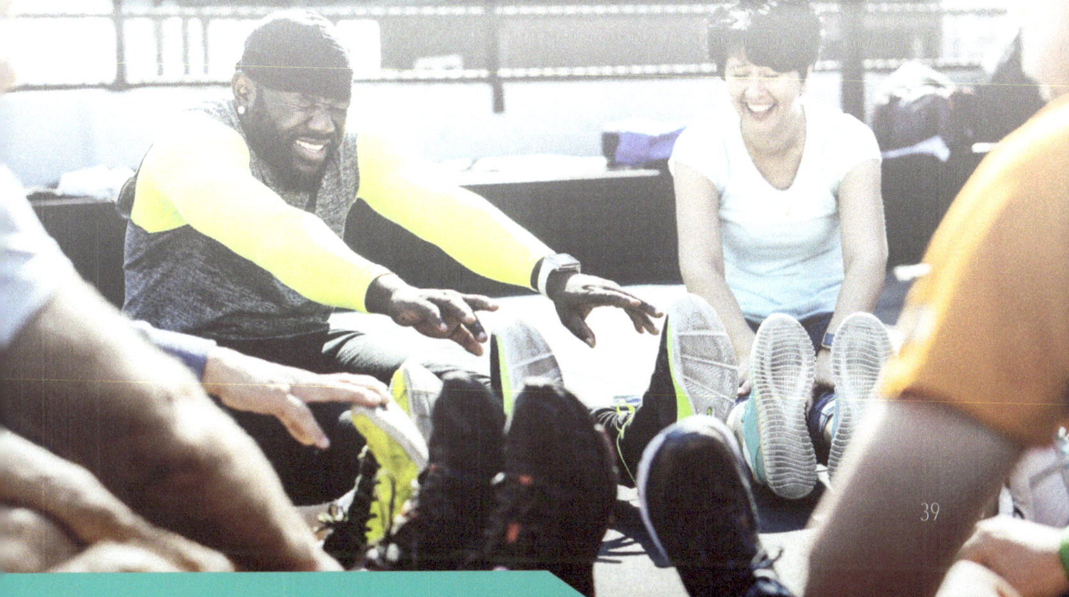

THE BUSY PROFESSIONAL BLUEPRINT COACHING ACADEMY

Are you overweight? Do you feel unhealthy? Are you overwhelmed and stressed and have a hard time getting it all done? Do you feel tired, lethargic and depressed? Do you lack time? Are you inconsistent with your workouts or lack the knowledge to get the results you'd like? If you said yes to

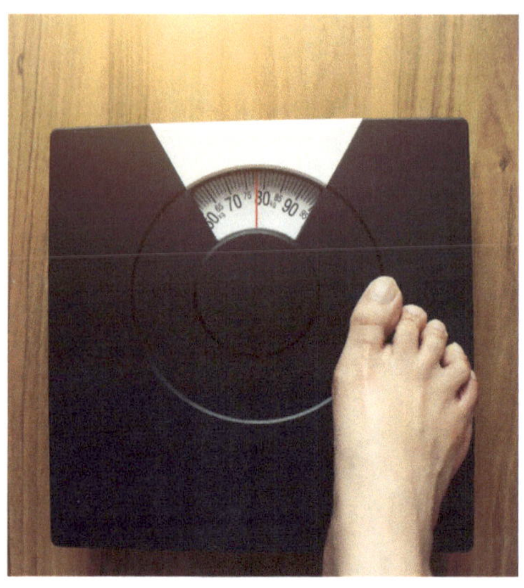

any of these questions then we have the solution to your problem. It's time for a change, a life altering change! Allow me to introduce you to The Busy Professional Blueprint Academy. An exclusive online coaching program for Busy Professionals who would like to take their health to the next level. We possess the solution to your problems…

If chosen you must be willing to put in the time, work and effort to become the very best version of yourself. The process isn't easy but as you already know nothing worth having never is… During your time with us you will not only learn how to workout more effectively but you will learn how to eat to maximize health and get leaner while simultaneously "bullet proofing" your body with cutting edge recovery techniques to reduce pain and prevent injury.

You will no longer be the same person!

Your mind, sharp and clear from distraction and you will possess laser like focus. You will possess the strength, vigor and stamina of your High School days and be ready to crush your day. You will lose weight, be leaner, toner, healthier and have the tools to manage your daily stress. Your joints will be healthy, lubricated and free from pain, moving like a gazelle. You will walk taller exuding the confidence to tackle any job or task. You will become the absolute best version of yourself! We will literally give you the blueprint to success.

APPLY HERE FOR ONLINE COACHING NOW:
primalfit360miami.com/online-coaching/

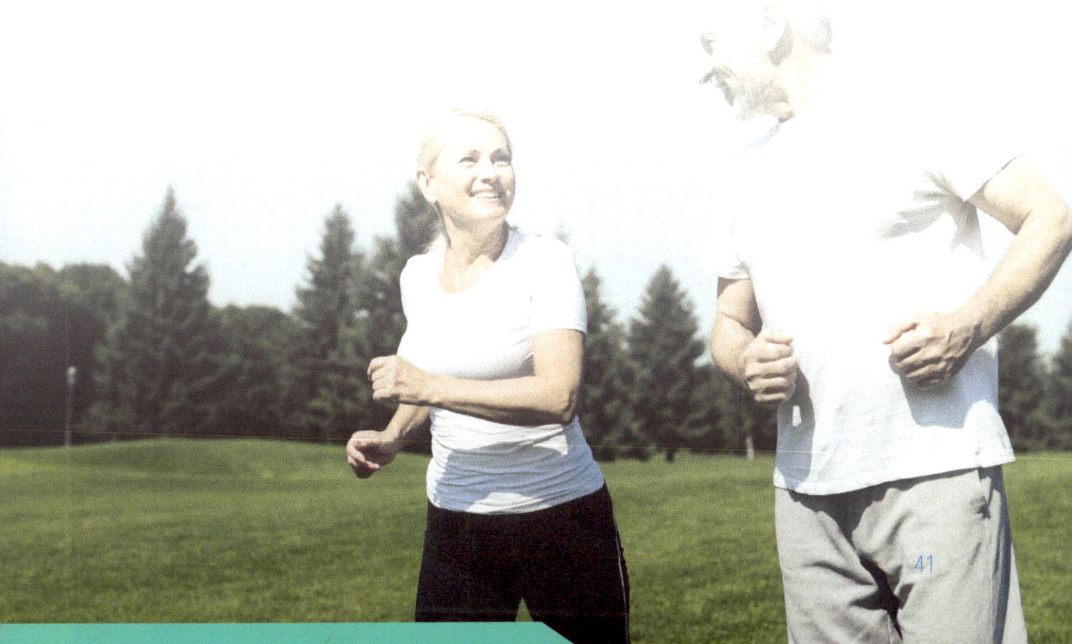

30 DAY CHALLENGE TESTIMONIALS:

So tonight I got to see myself on camera; specifically for an video interview I did back on May 25th. I couldn't look at it. I was 18ibs heavier and my face was so swollen and full. I am now certain more than ever that the "FAST PACK" program works for me and watching this video has motivated me to keep going until I reach a weigh that brings me peace. Thank You Matt Pack for your guidance, support and genuine care. Ready for round two...

—Mary Rogers

Yesterday I went to a friends party and for the first time ever I wore a crop top and I felt amazing.

Never been comfortable enough to do that before!!

—Scarlett Hernandez

I lost 35 pounds since May, (which included 2 vacations), I no longer have heartburn nor any digestive issues. I now fit into all my clothes except one pair of pants.

I no longer use food for comfort, I also know that I can skip a meal and won't die of hunger. I do not have any 3 o'clock cravings for sweets. I lost all my sugar addictions.

For the first time I KNOW, I am in full control of my eating. The fasting lifestyle will be with me forever.

Matt Pack thank you for the best tool you've ever given me and you have given me many.

—Gloria Del Valle Wilder

I'm 24 lbs down in one month and feeling very happy to have accomplished my goal by my 30th Bday this Saturday. I've learned a lot and am very thankful by everyone's help in this group!

—Joshua Riddle

Damn it's 30 days already?

It was a lot easier than I thought it could ever be.

I stumbled a few times but got back up, kept going and dropped 29 pounds!!

Thanks for all your support Matt Pack and everyone in the group. My journey has just begun…

—Jason Thorstensen

I was able to complete my 30 days in July and I lost 18lbs. but The most positive impacts for me was the support from everyone around me including my Fast Pack family, accountability, recognizing my strengths/weaknesses and the motivation.

I see my self excelling to my goal and if I mess up I have the tools to use to get back on track.

*From the words of my dear leader… "F**k being realistic" I'm driving this in full gear.*

—Ericka HisLady Jenrette

I did the challenge in July and lost 10 pounds. I traveled A LOT!!! I believe my attitude towards meals, snacking at parties and pressure from others to eat or drink has completely changed.

—Jennifer Romanik Geimer

I lost 20 lbs in the 30 day challenge but the most positive thing is seeing that I could actually lose stubborn fat, esp. in my stomach!

—Bonnie Pack

This entire experience has changed my association with food. The way I perceived it and used it was not really healthy.

In the past Food had a very emotional role. I would crave a donut enjoy it for 5 mins and then hate myself for two days.

Knowing it's ok to indulge as long as it's balanced to the rest of your intake was an important lesson for me.

I feel less emotional and more rational about my food choices now than I did at the beginning.

I've also learned to stand up for my health!

This one I merit to this amazing group. I didn't realize how much of an influence people have on your eating. So figuring out ways not to be influenced by others, specially family, was a HUGE accomplishment for me.

I can honestly say that I feel like I can enjoy what I like, keep a healthy lifestyle, and keep my weight where I want it!

Karen Matamoros

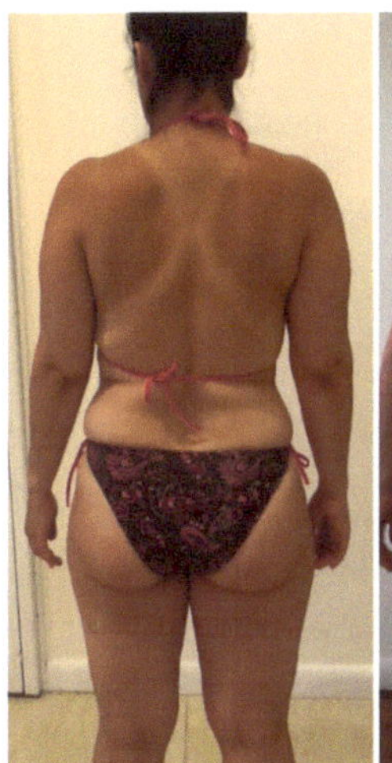
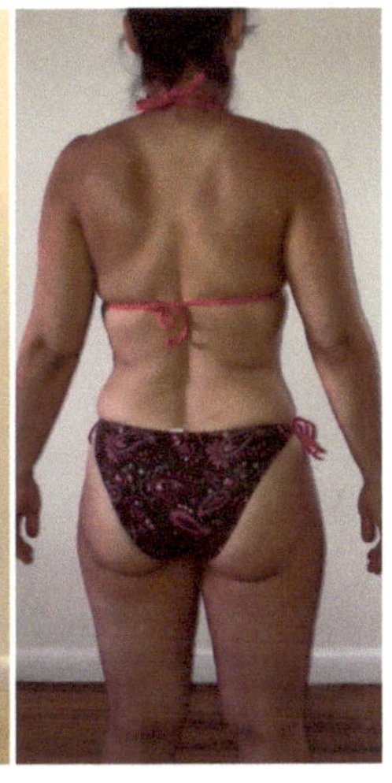
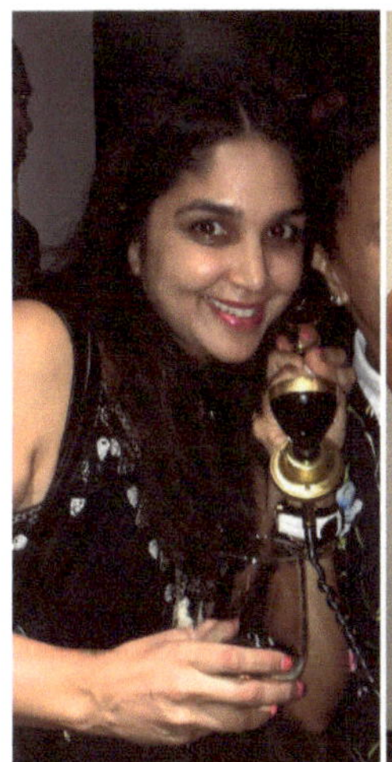
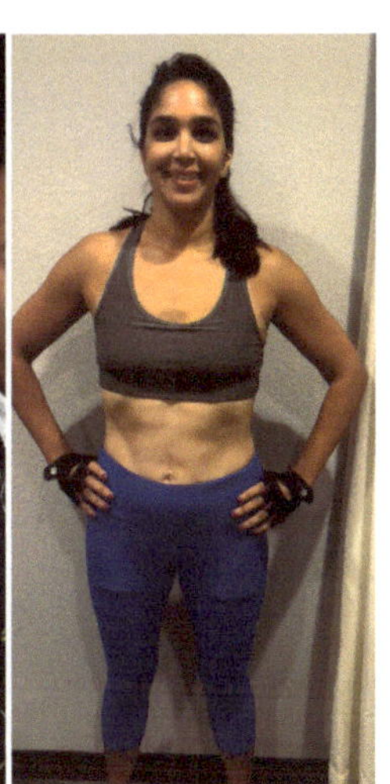
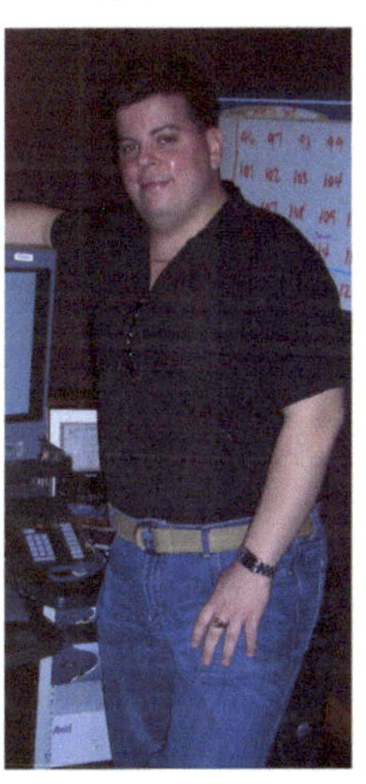
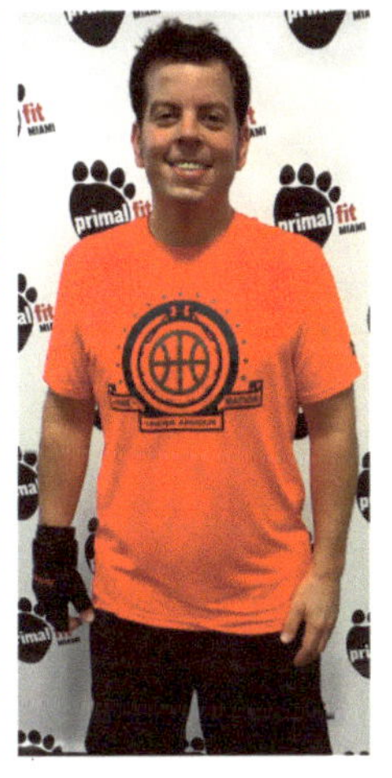
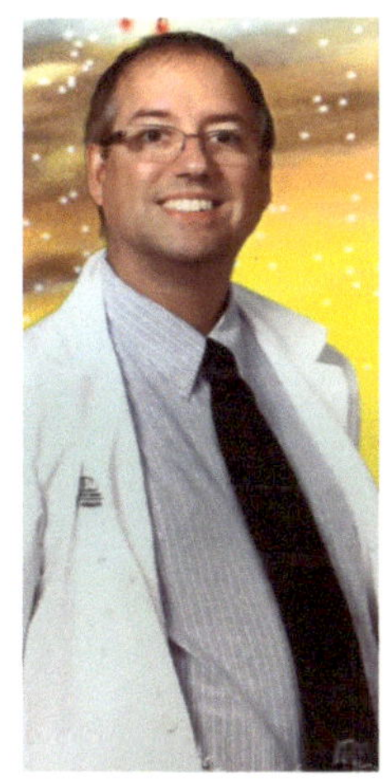
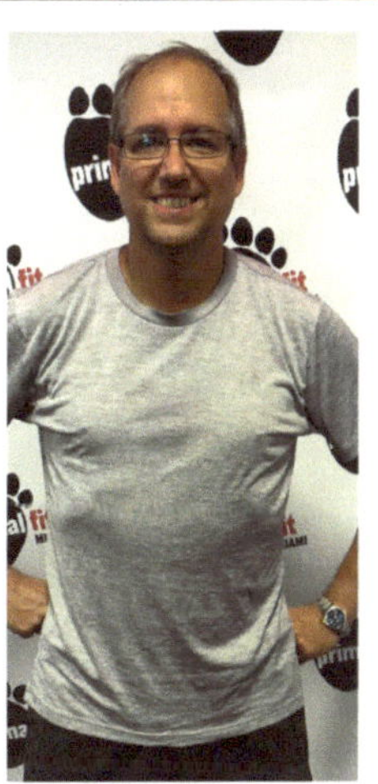
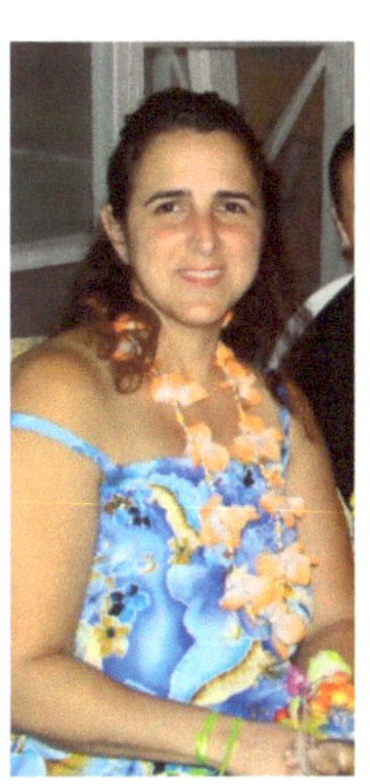
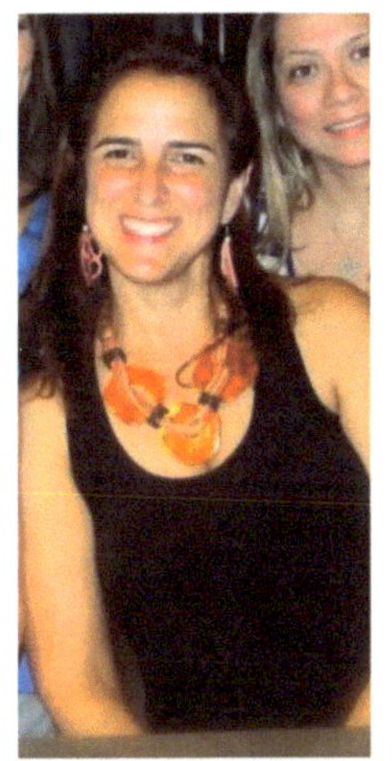
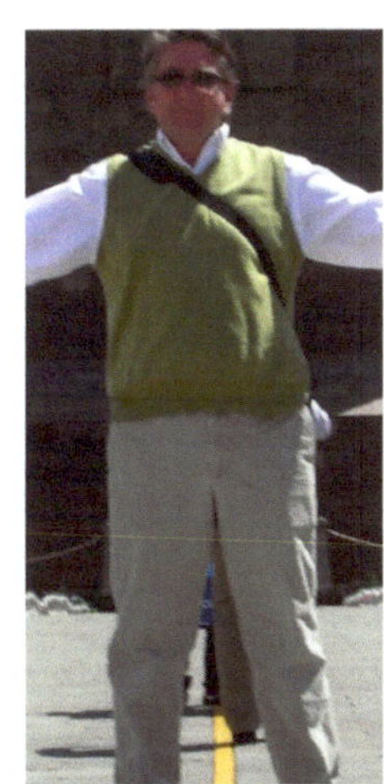
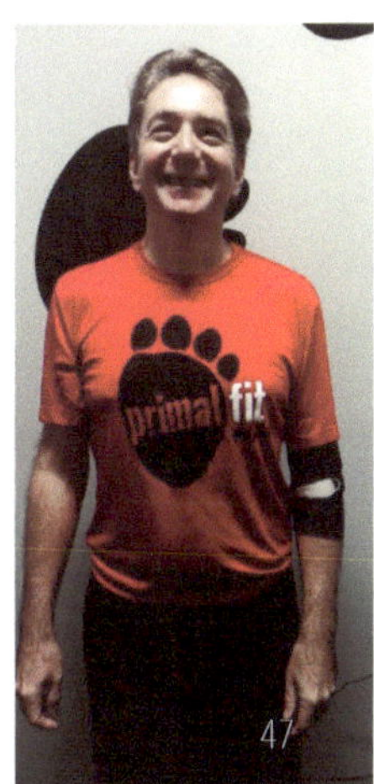

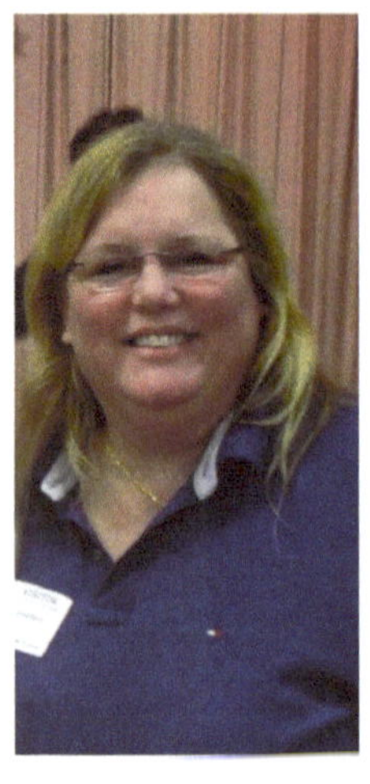
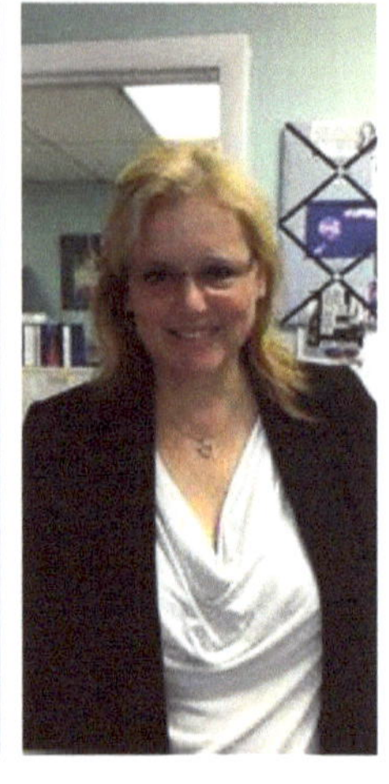
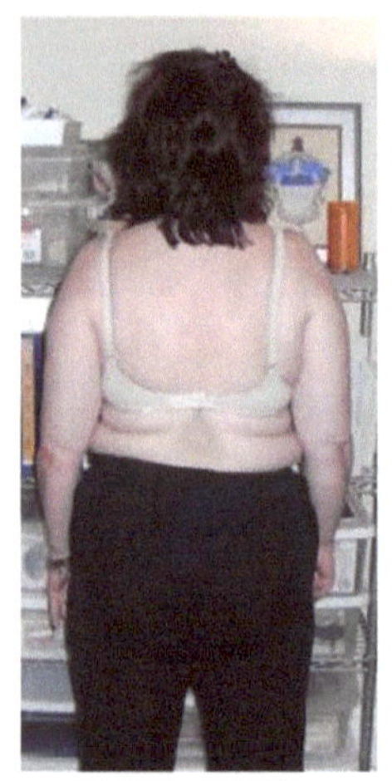
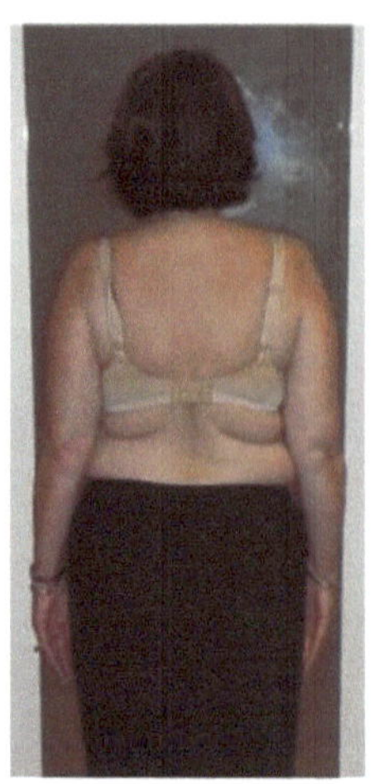
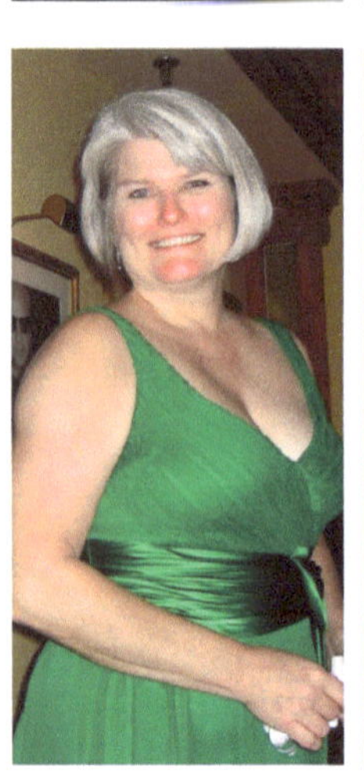
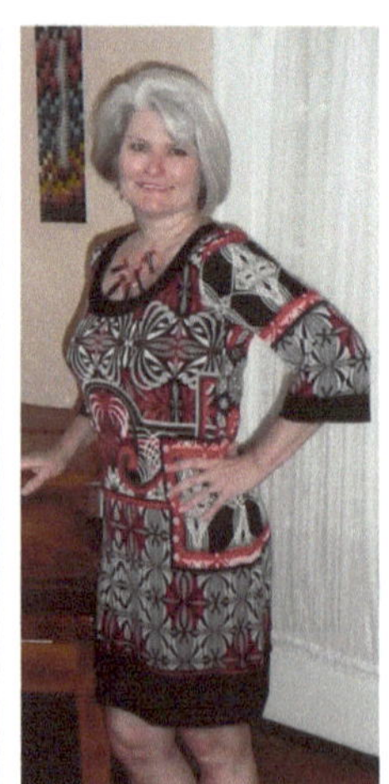
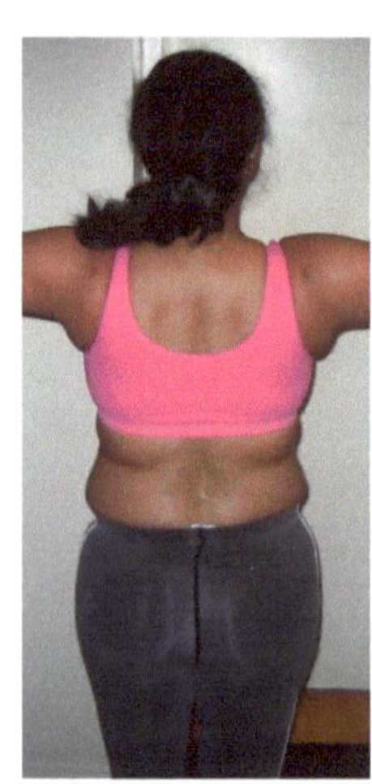
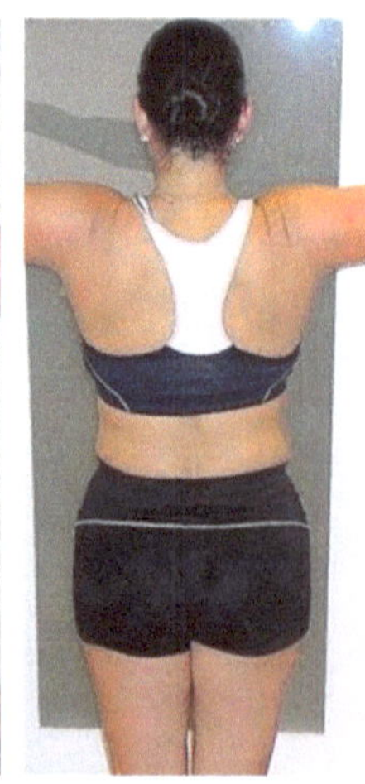
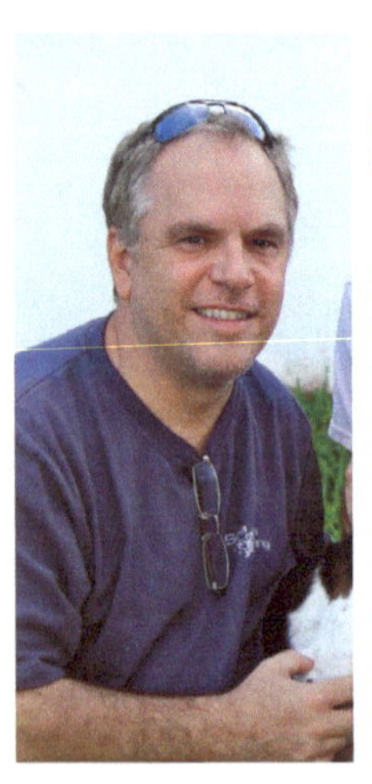
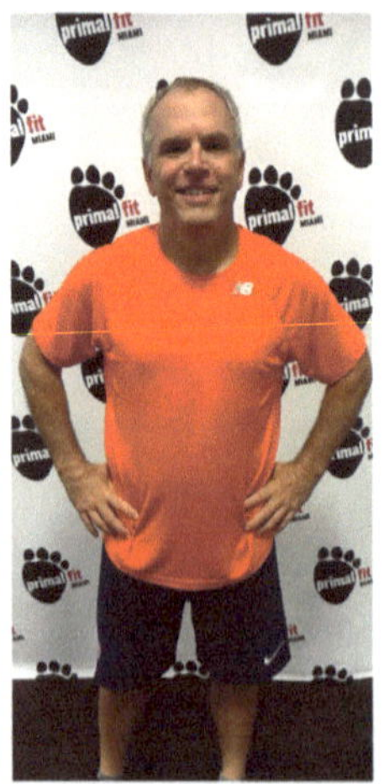
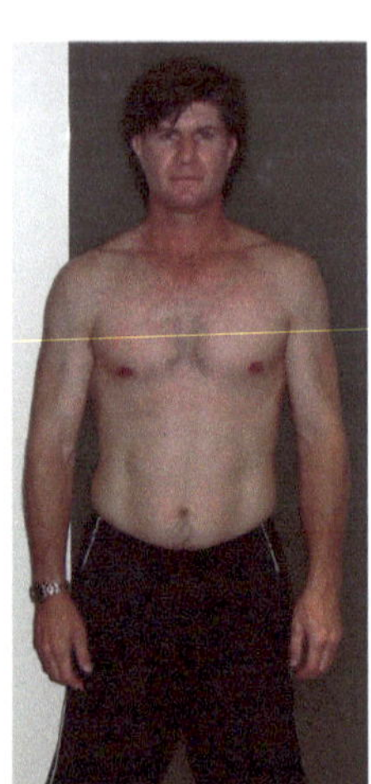
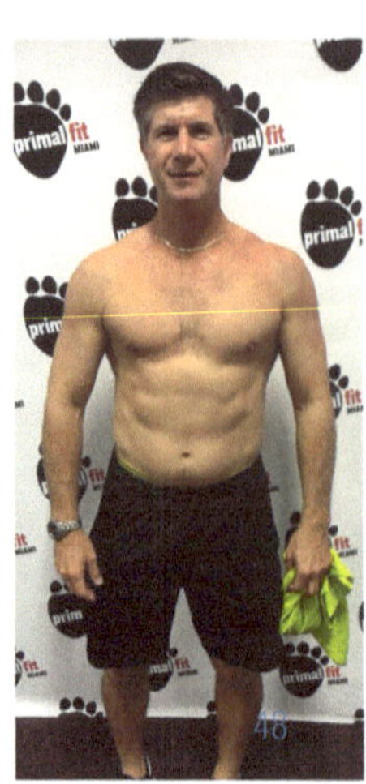

BEFORE & AFTER

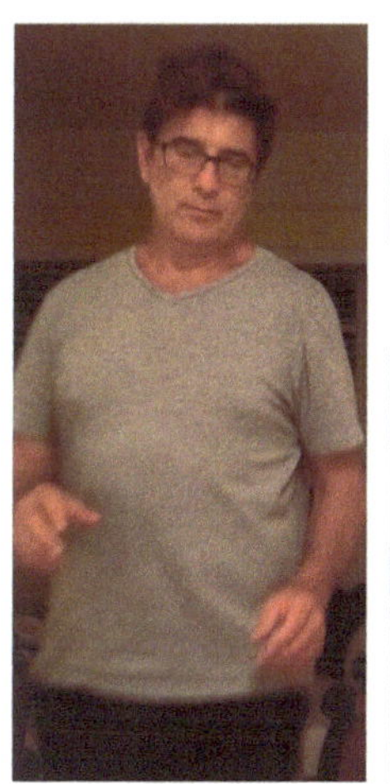 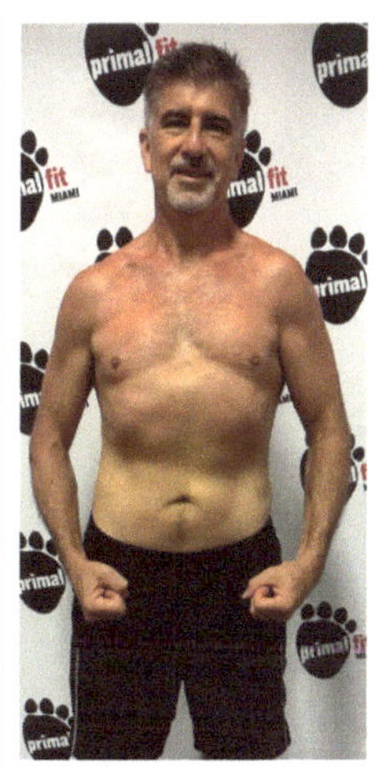 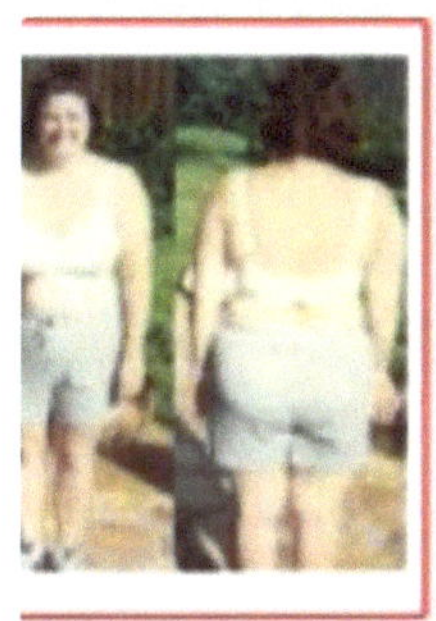 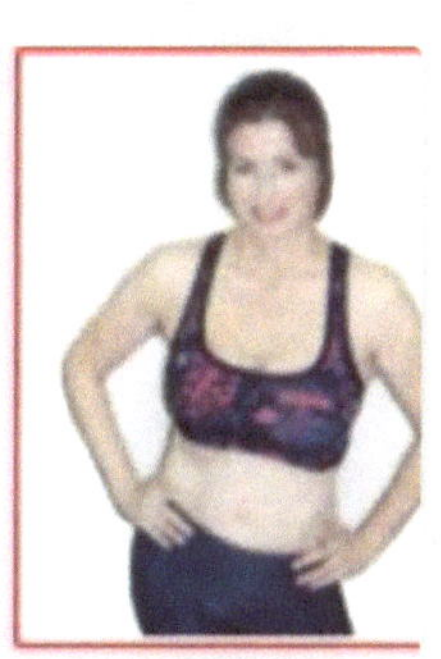
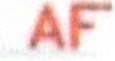
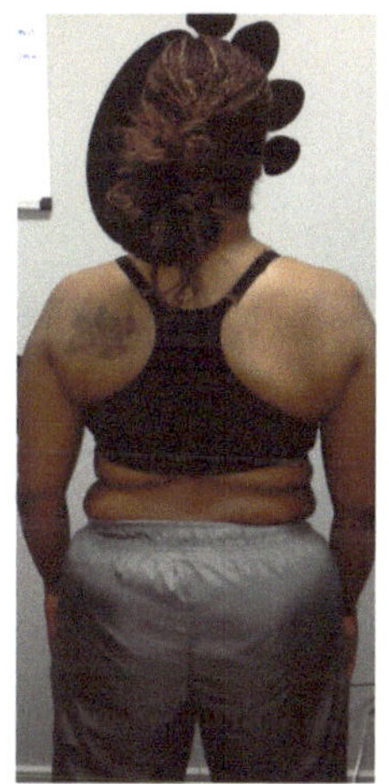 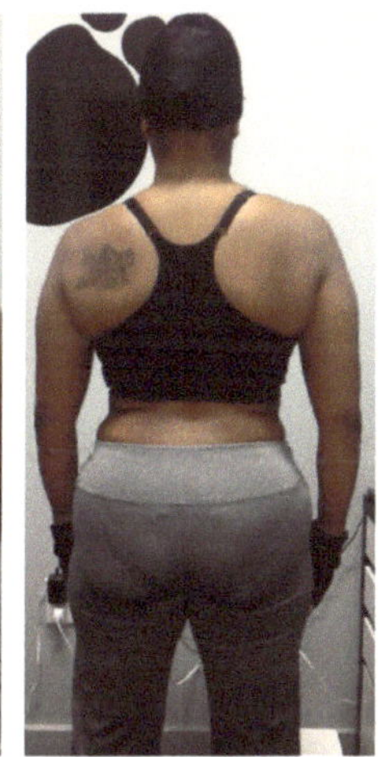 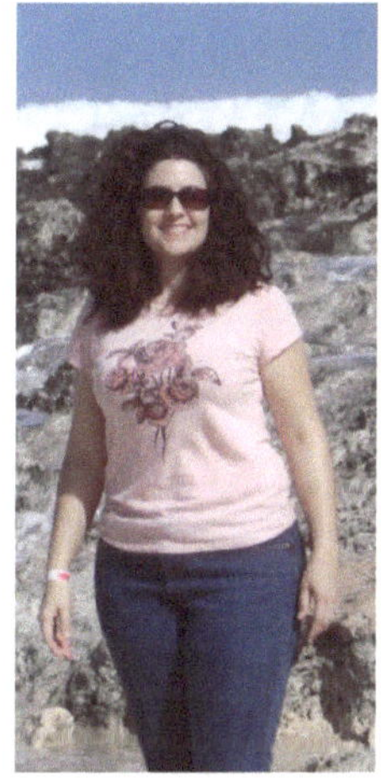 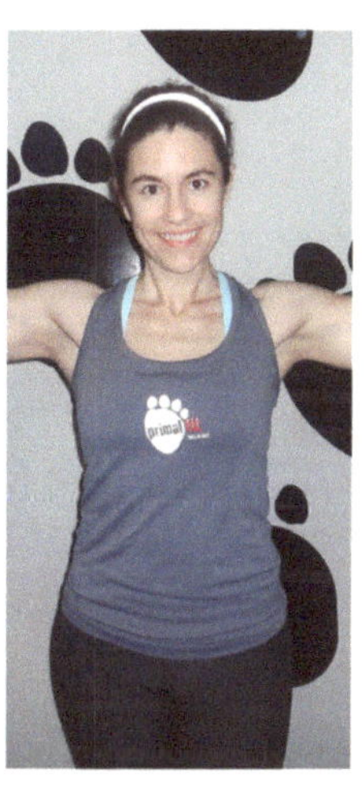
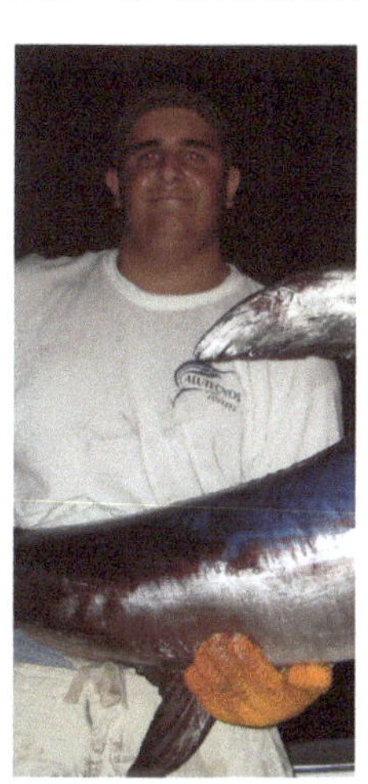 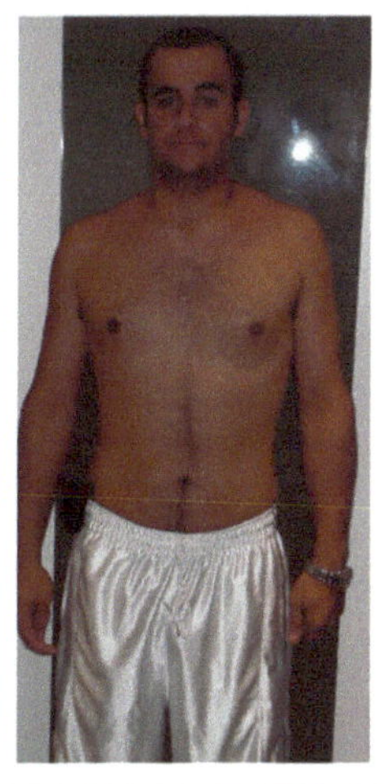 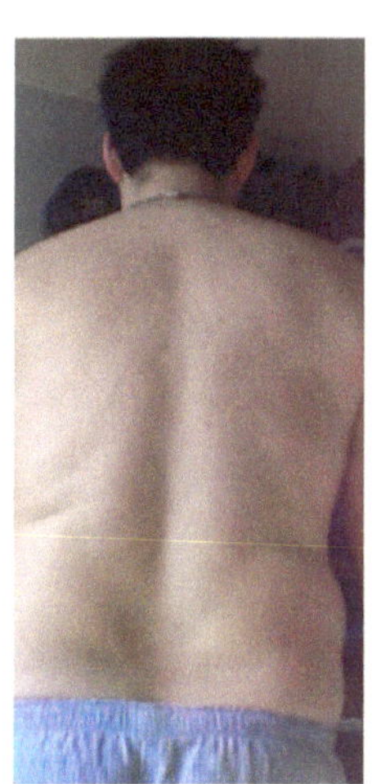 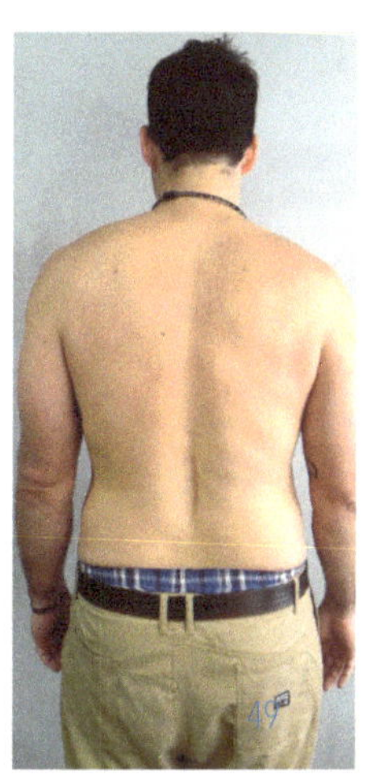

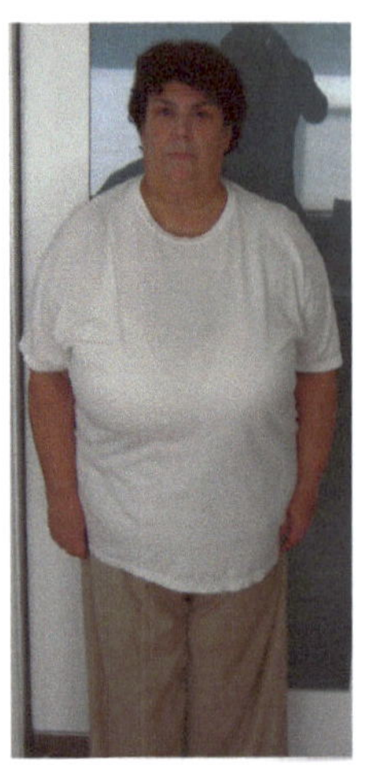
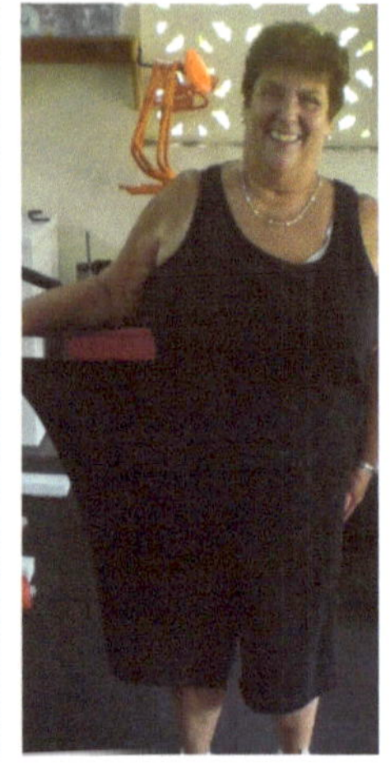
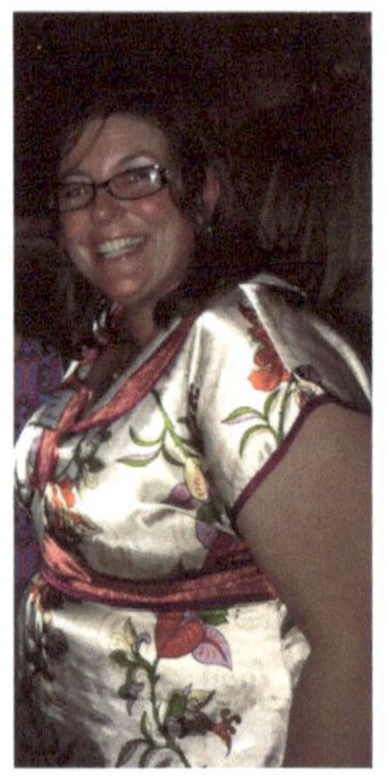
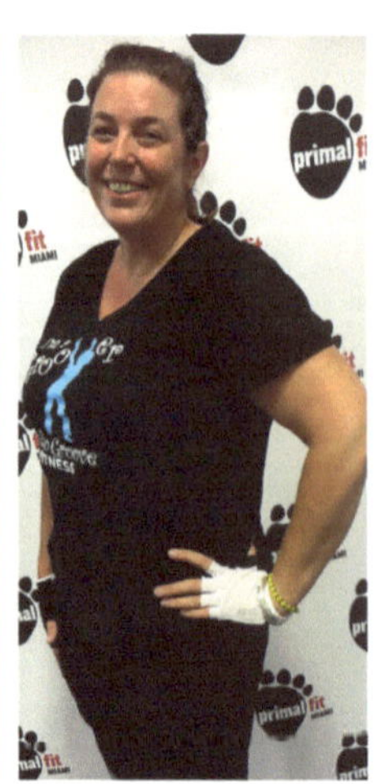
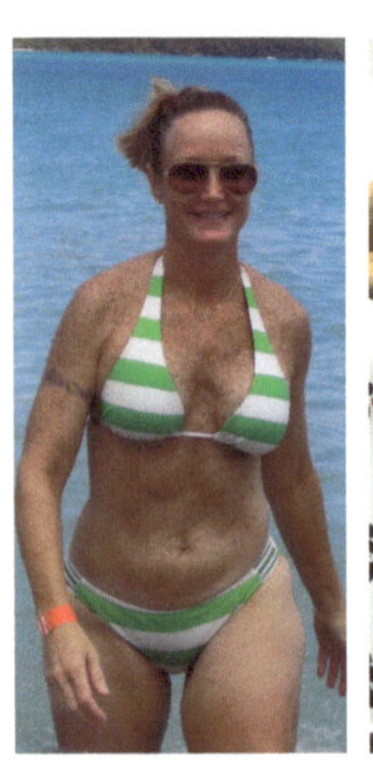
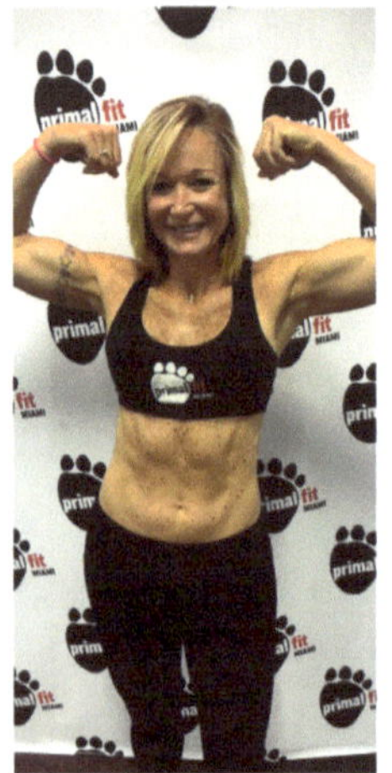
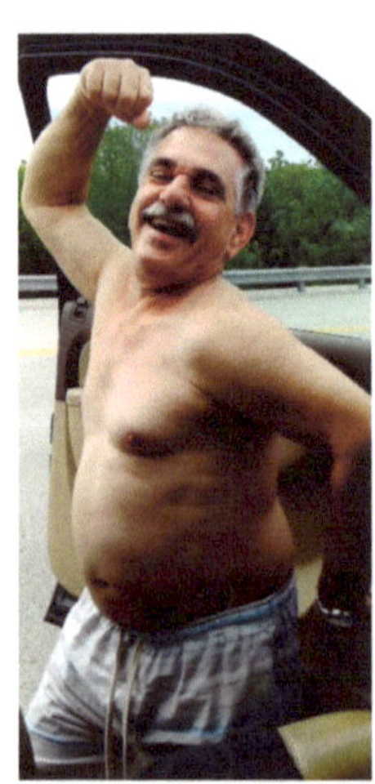
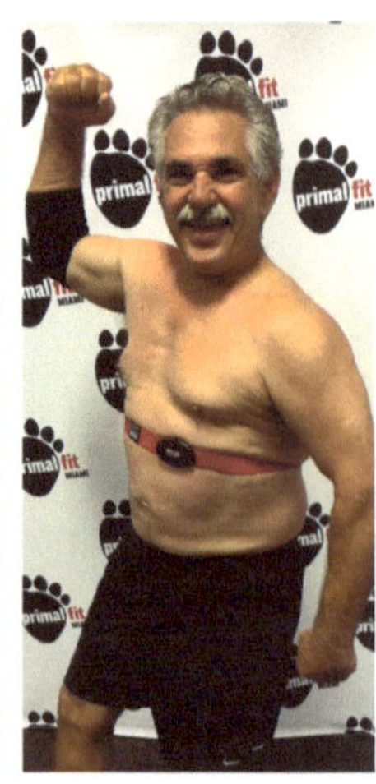
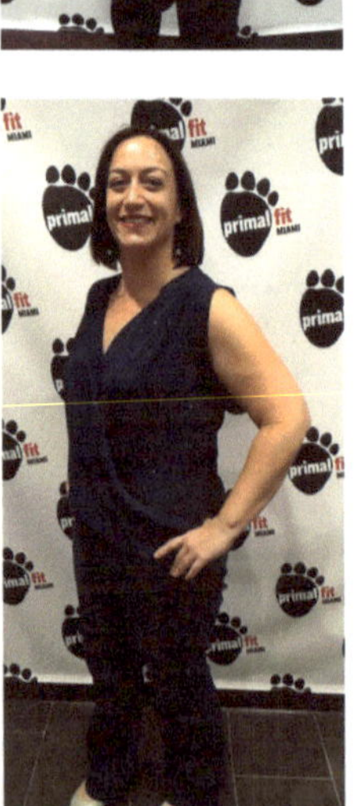
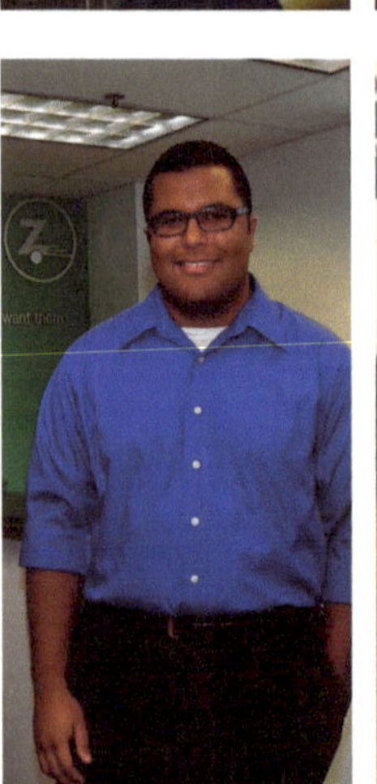
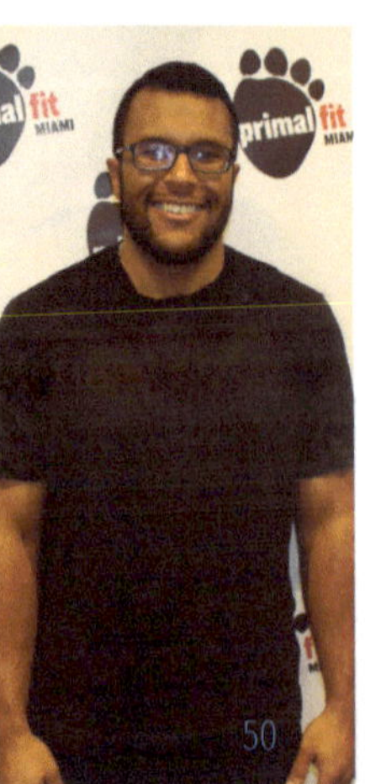

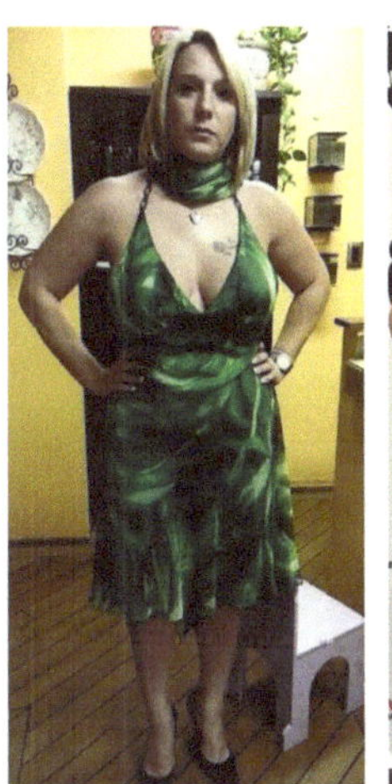
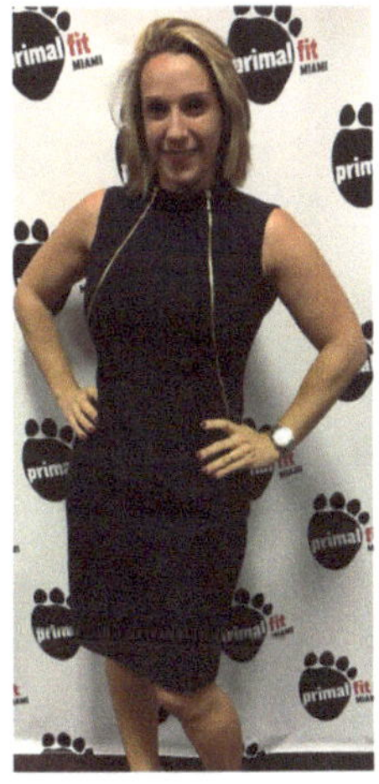
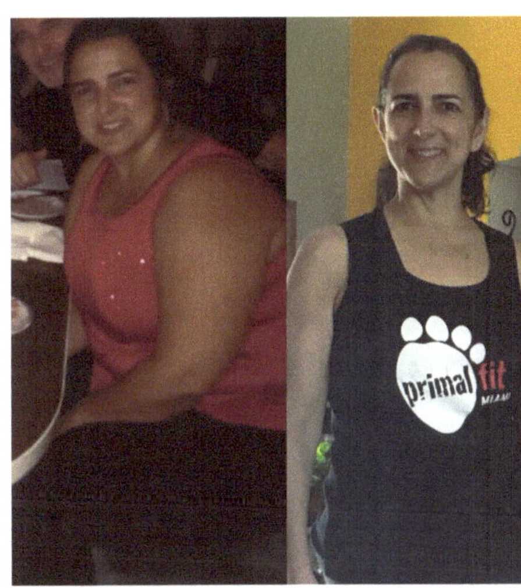
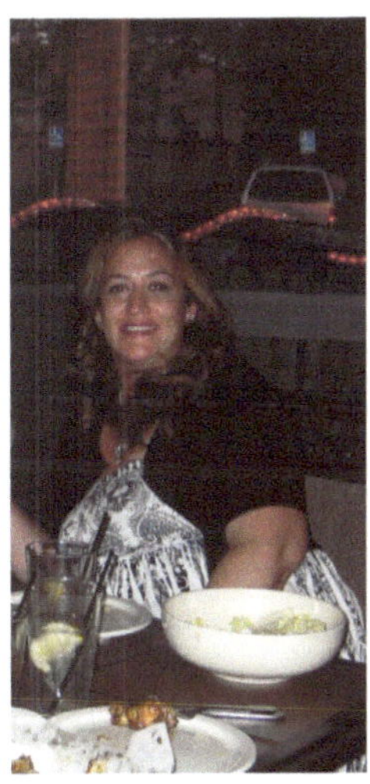
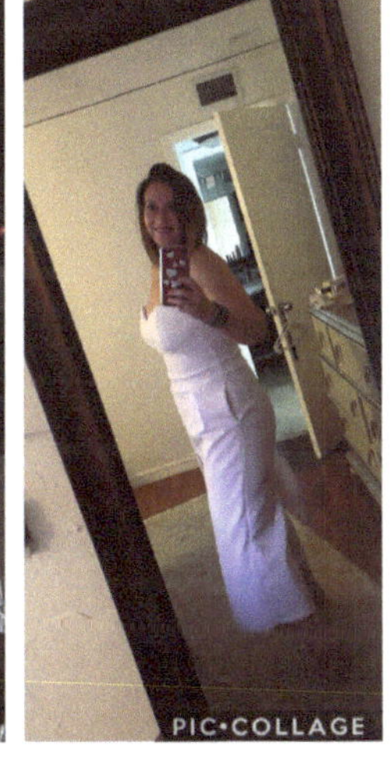
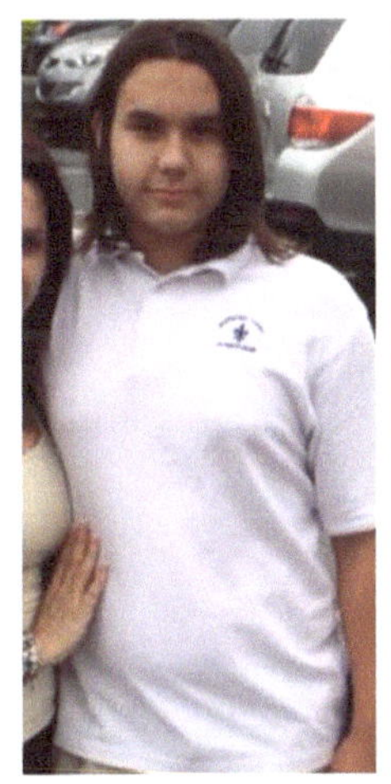
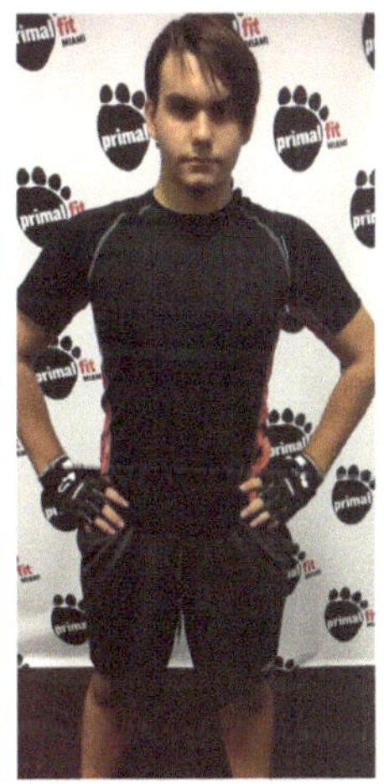
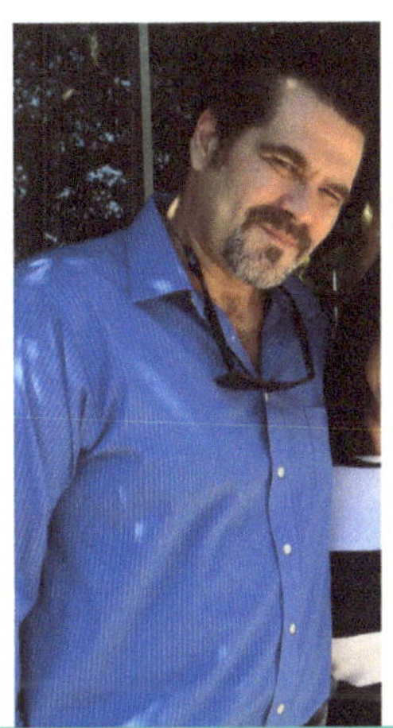
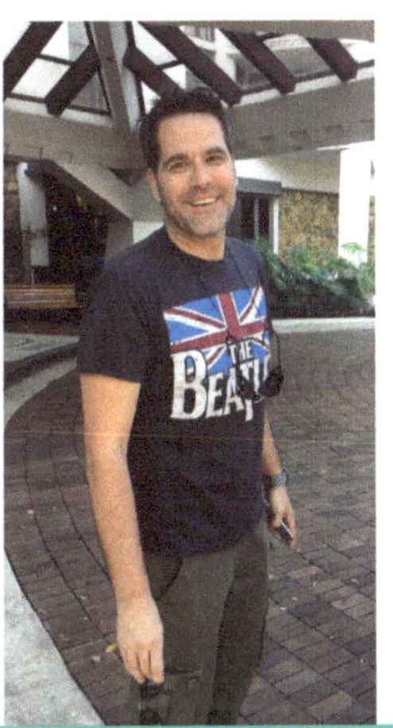
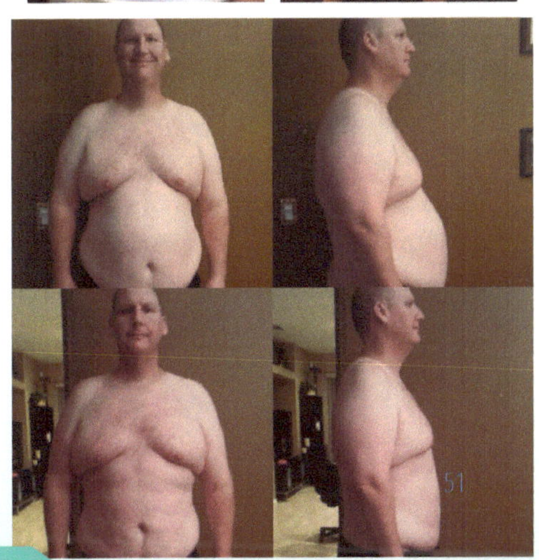

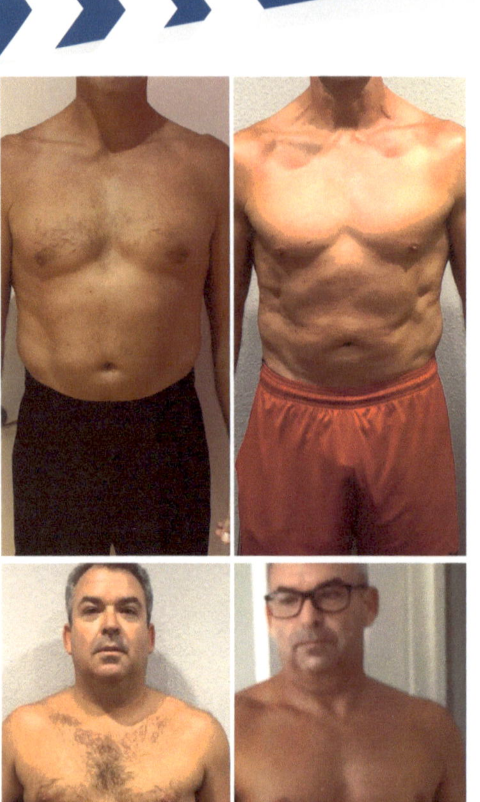
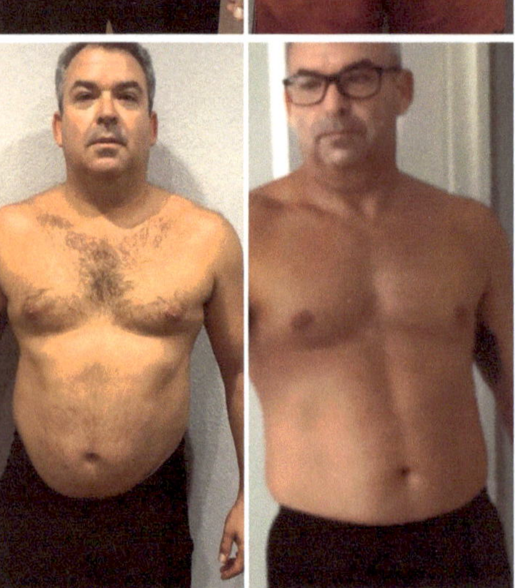
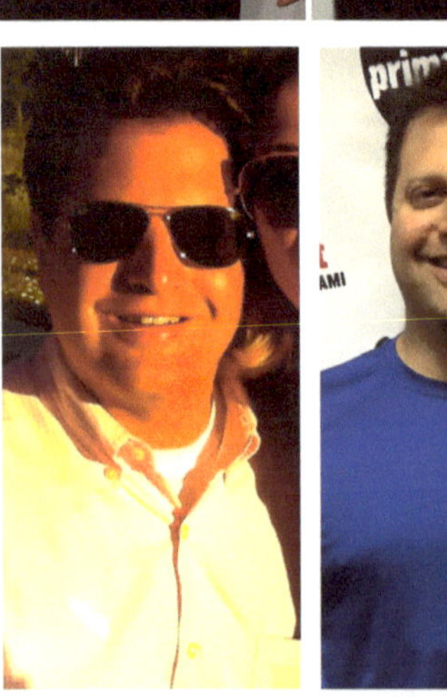
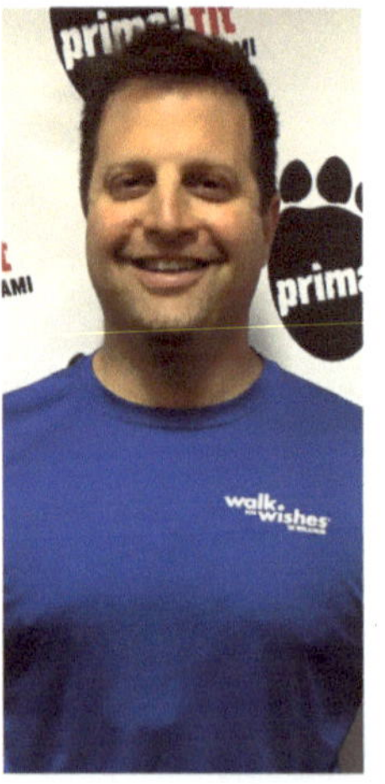
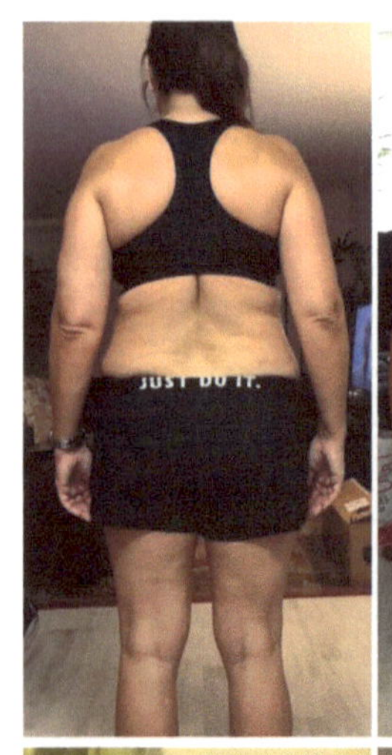
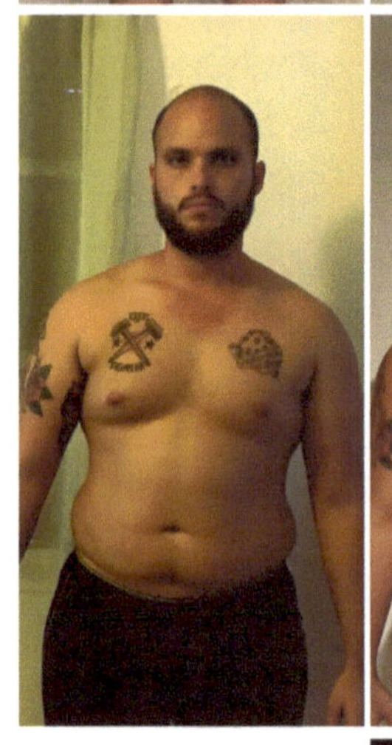
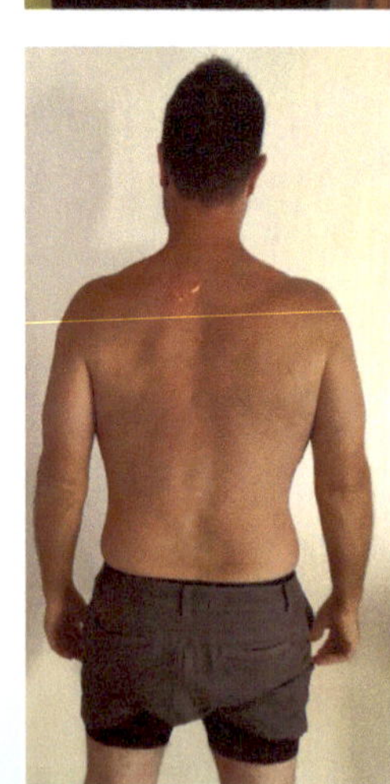
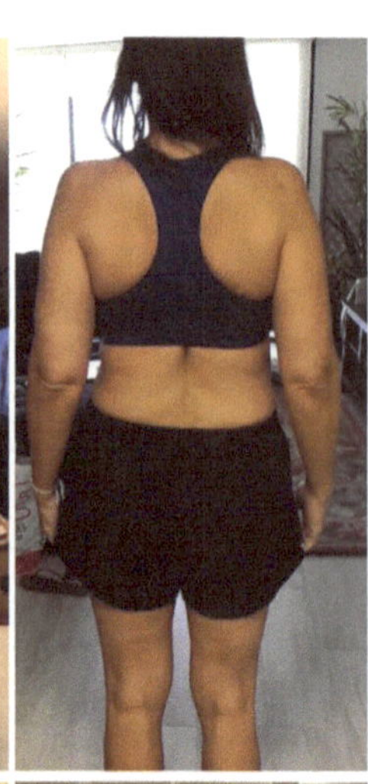
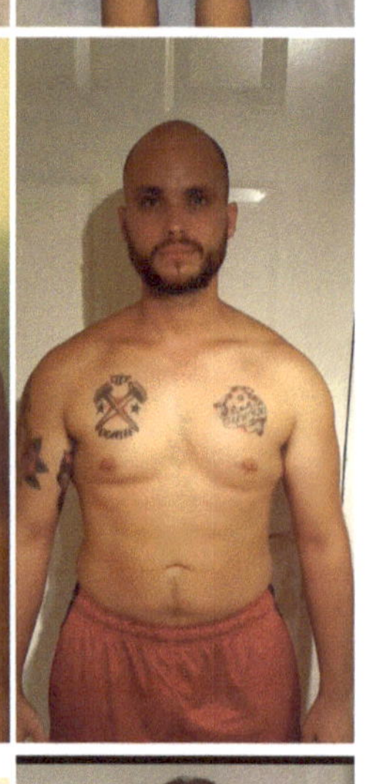
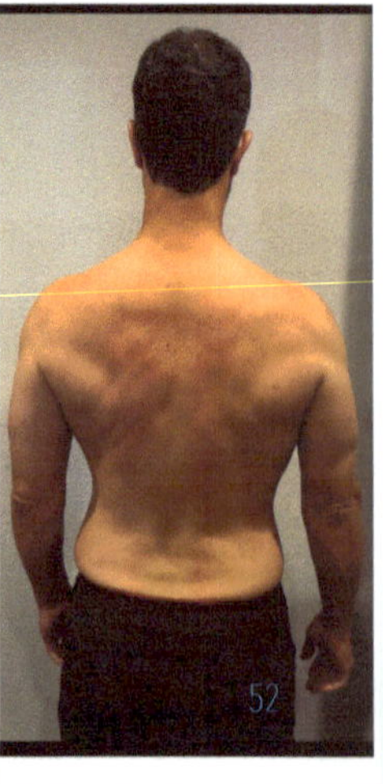

BEFORE & AFTER

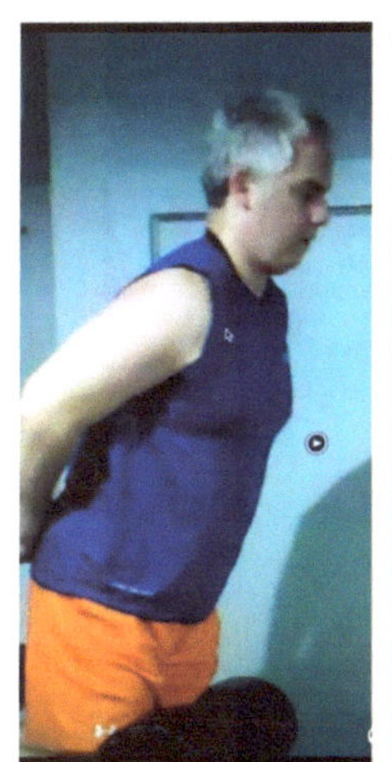 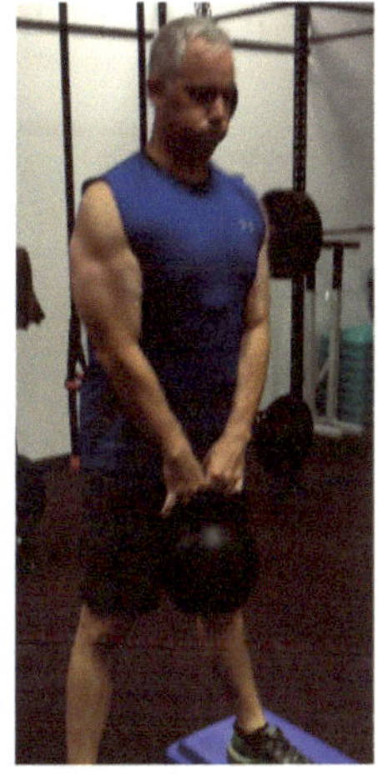 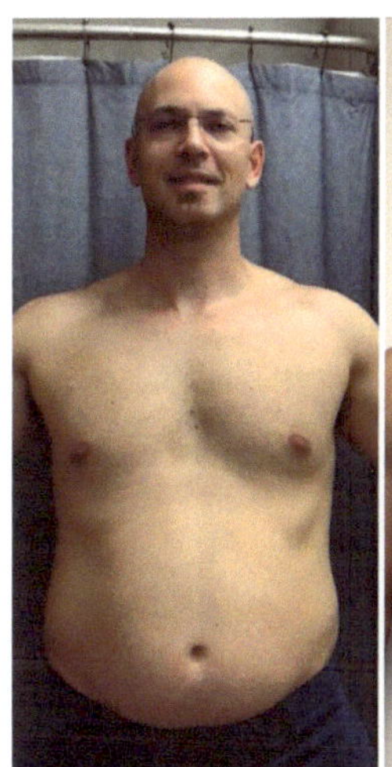 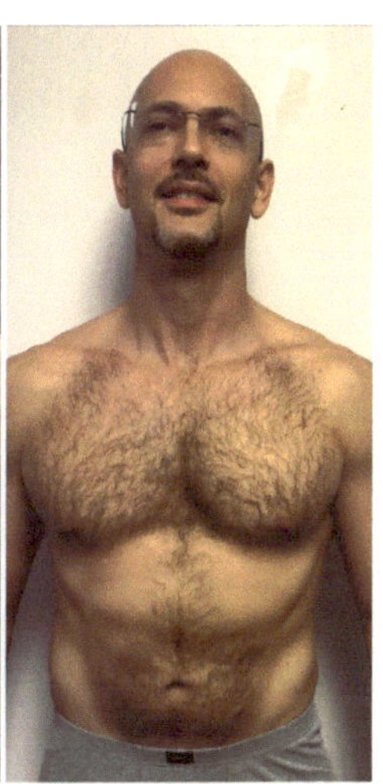

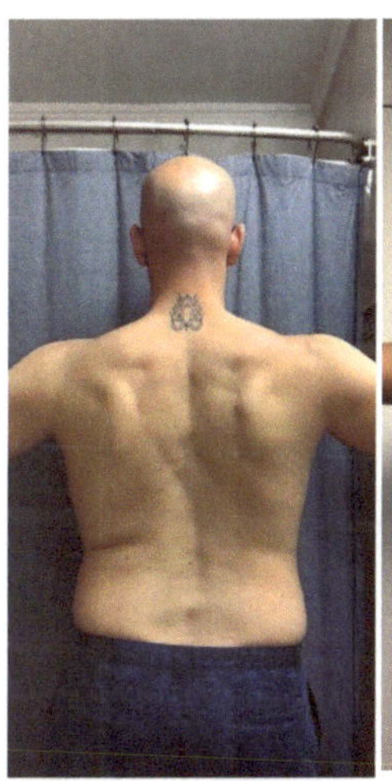 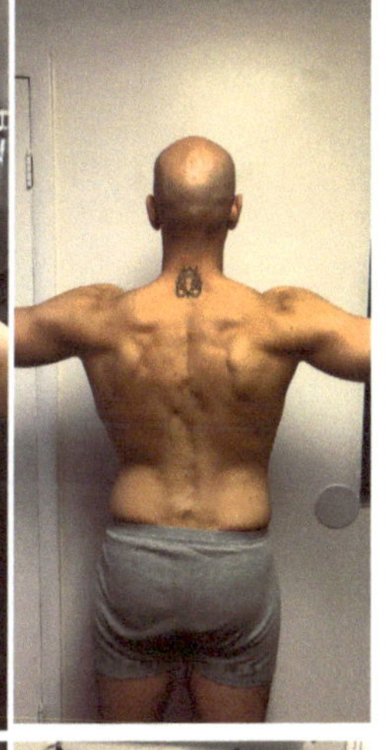 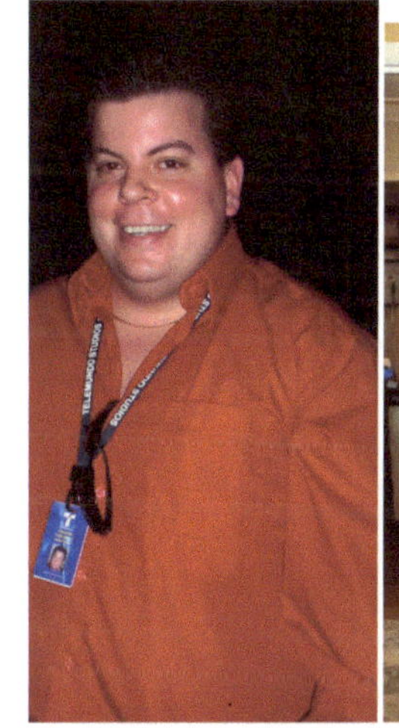 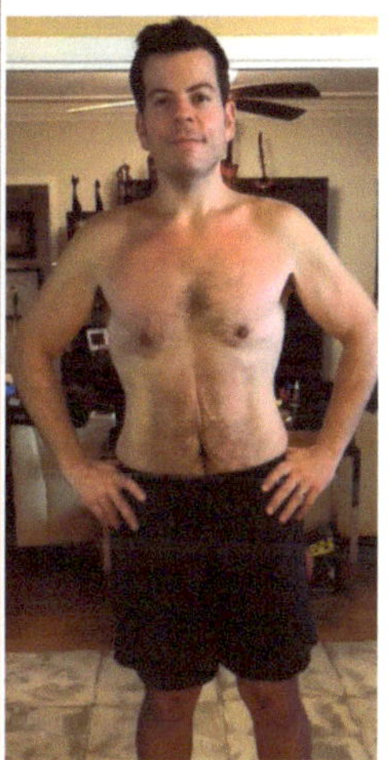

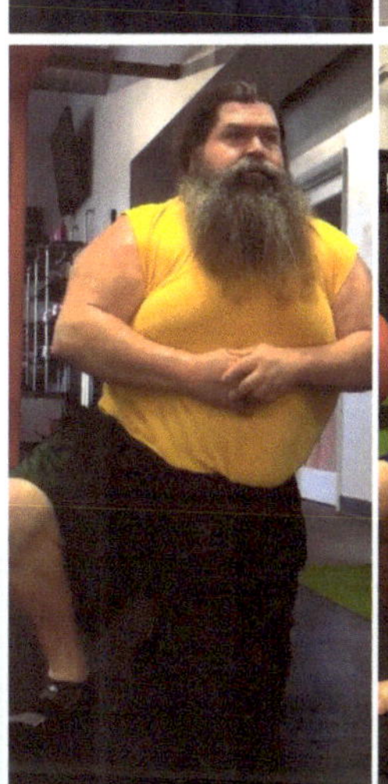 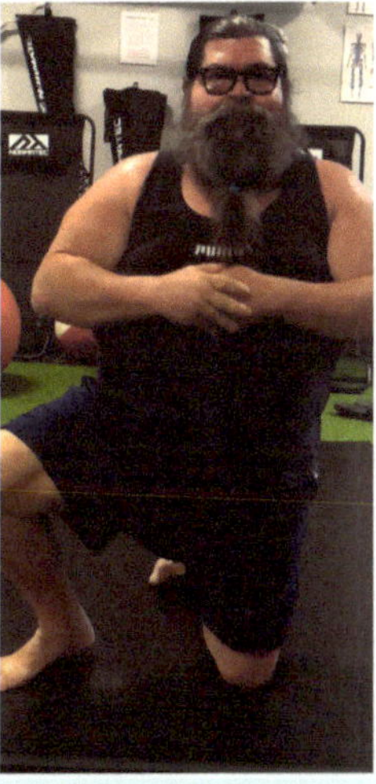 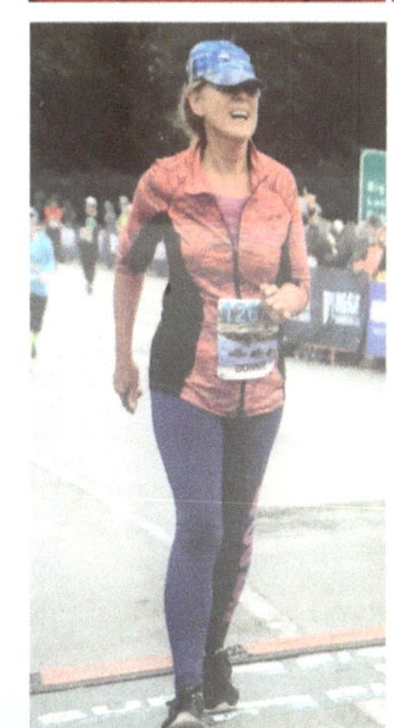 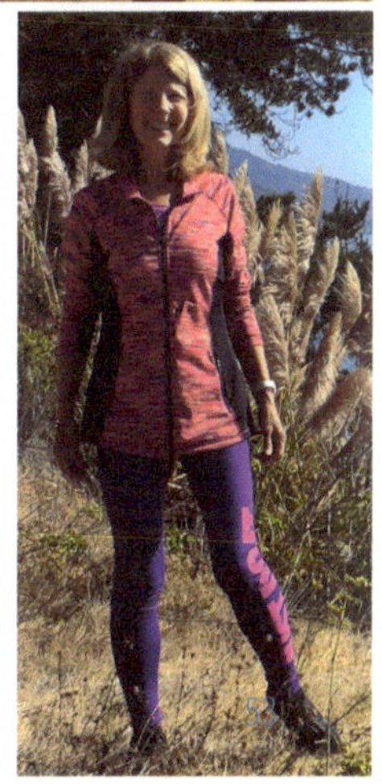